AUTOBIOGRAPHY OF NURSE KNOWLES:

The Experiences of a Nurse in Training in Liverpool, 1928–1931

Written by
E A Mclaughlin

from the recollections of
Mrs F E Creswell

MINERVA PRESS

LONDON

MONTREUX   LOS ANGELES   SYDNEY

AUTOBIOGRAPHY OF NURSE KNOWLES:

The Experiences of a Nurse in Training in Liverpool, 1928–1931

To the memory of the many colleagues with whom I shared this training and especially all my students male and female with whom I spent the happiest days of my life and whom now I consider to be my friends.

Sadly Auntie Eva (Nurse Knowles) passed away before she was able to see her book in print. It is in her fond memory and with much love and respect that this book is published.

Mrs Creswell's fund of memories of a time and style of training now lost to us is so informative and amusing, thought-provoking and entertaining, that a book of those memories was simply asking to be written. To form a coherent story from the isolated incidents she recollects seemed the best way to bring her lively personality to life.

Nurse Knowles (as she was then) went on to further training as a midwife and fever nurse and then continued her career in various hospitals in the North West area up to, during, and after the Second World War. She was a teaching sister for over 25 years and retired in 1963. Over 1,000 students passed their finals under her expert tutelage.

She still keeps in touch with many people; pupils, colleagues and patients as well, and is held in great affection by all. She is now eighty-eight. Over the years several people have told her that she should record her stories, and at her annual reunion with some of her pupils the news that she was providing the material for a book was greeted with enthusiasm.

Foreword

by Mrs F E Creswell SRN, SCM, SRFN, BTA(Hons), HC, NT Cert.

To my readers – some I may know, some I have taught, and some unknown to me – I wish and hope you enjoy reading of my experiences in the early nursing years of my life.

I would like to thank Mrs Liz McLaughlin for her help and encouragement, making this possible for me.

I have not mentioned anyone by name but some may recognise events shared with me. The Royal Southern Hospital is no longer in use, but the nurses are now part of the huge Liverpool General Hospital.

They were happy days; hard work, great comradeship, and well worth while.

Contents

Arrival

On a warm day in late May of the year 1928 I was walking purposefully down Liverpool's Hill Street, carrying a suitcase, until I reached the Royal Southern Hospital. I put my suitcase down at my feet for a moment and looked up. Set alongside the terraced houses, the hospital was a large, imposing building on four floors. Three broad stone steps led to the pillared doorway. I checked my watch. The time was fifteen minutes to three, I was in good time for my appointment. I picked up my suitcase again and walked up the steps and into the hall.

There was a porter's room just to the left of the entrance and a uniformed porter looked out to see if I needed any help.

"Miss Knowles," I told him, "to start my training."

He nodded, indicated a bench in the hall and returned to his post.

I moved across to join the two other girls who were already sitting in the hallway with a suitcase and a bundle at their feet. By the time three o'clock came there were six of us waiting. After smiling at each other and introducing ourselves, we fell quiet (apart from one girl, a little older than the rest of us, who told us that she had already done a years training at an Eye Hospital). I was free to reflect on the decisions that had led her here. How simple to want to be a nurse, how prolonged the preparations had seemed to be.

Months and months ago, the nurse who had come to look after Grandma when she had pneumonia had impressed me deeply with her kindness. She had been so efficient and so caring in her work. While she tended the old lady in what was to be her final illness the nurse had often talked to me about it and I began to be drawn to the idea of nursing as a career for myself. I loved working with people, I was not afraid of hard work, nor squeamish about the sick, and all in all it seemed to me that I had found something I really wanted to do.

I was the eldest daughter of four in the family. I had no wish to burden my parents any further by taking an expensive training course, but this consideration, which had held me back from a tentative plan to study Physical Culture at Bedford College, was swept away when I found out that the cost of a nurse's training was comparatively small. Once this point had been settled for me (and a good deal of encouragement given to me as well) by Grandmother's nurse, I went to my parents and told them what I wanted to do.

"Enrol on a three year training course to be a nurse?" they said.

"I'll give you three months before you give up," said my father.

"Six months before you come home again," said my mother.

That seemed to be the only point on which they disagreed – how long it would be before I arrived back on the doorstep, beaten.

(Years later, I realised that they had both known exactly what such a challenge would do to me. Their apparent scepticism had been just what I needed to make me stick to my decision like glue. Whatever they thought about it in reality, their seeming to doubt me did not stop them from helping me at any rate.)

The first thing I had to do was to write to various teaching hospitals to see if they would take me on. This was not how I thought of it though. I was quite unaware of any possibility of difficulty and I expected such a rush for my services when it was known that I was available, that I told the family I was sending four letters to four hospitals and whichever one replied first would be the lucky hospital to get me. Then I settled down to wait for the answers.

Thankfully I was not picked by any of them. In fact, with parental guidance and advice from others, I had settled on Lancaster Royal Infirmary, Preston Royal Infirmary, Liverpool Royal Infirmary, and the Royal Southern Hospital at Liverpool as my choices. They were all good teaching hospitals and within reasonable distance from home; because I would be living in this was vital to me for days off and visiting.

As it happened, it was the Royal Southern that replied first to my letter and replied indeed, with such a lot of queries and requests that I was startled to discover I had more to do than just politely accept their invitation. There were forms to fill in and references to be obtained before I was even properly offered a place! The doctor and the minister were approached and proved happy to vouch for me being a suitable young lady, and my school certificates bore witness to my ability to learn. When all the information requested had been sent back, there was another period of waiting to go through until the day the letter accepting me for training arrived.

With it came a further batch of things to do, but I felt that at least it was a step in the right direction because all of these things were related to actually getting ready to start my training.

There was a list of uniform – three dresses (purple check), twelve aprons (twelve!), separate collars and cuffs for the dresses, black stockings and black shoes with flat, rubber-tipped heels – and please bring your own fountain pen, scissors, watch, etc., etc., etc.

The address from which to purchase the uniform was also given – the Nursing Outfitting Association – and a shopping expedition was immediately planned. When I arrived with my mother at this huge emporium, I discovered that everything to do with the uniform was very strictly regulated. The dresses had to be exactly twelve inches from the ground, with three tucks around the skirt just above the hem. They were fitted in the bodice, with long sleeves and a full skirt. When I enquired why they came in the various different colours I could see hanging up along the racks, I found out that different hospitals, like different schools, had their own uniforms in their own colours. Throughout the nursing profession, however, sisters wore dark blue.

According to the list, the only thing the hospital provided for me would be the cap, everything else had to be paid for by my parents and brought with me when I reported to the hospital at 3 p.m. on my first day. So my parents paid for all the purchases and provided me with a suitcase to put them all in as well.

Then I waited again, marking time until the day the family went with me and my suitcase to Fleetwood Station to see me off.

So here I was on a warm day in late May of 1928, having travelled down by train to Liverpool and walked through the city to Hill Street; sitting with five other girls in the hall of the hospital, waiting once more, but I hoped for the last time, to begin my training as a nurse.

Idly, I looked along the hallway, noting the many doors on either side until my eyes came to rest on the huge full-length portrait of Prince Albert at the other end. The hall was a hundred and fifty yards long, but the picture was so big it was perfectly clear, even from where I was sitting at the front of the hospital.

The 'Royal' in Royal Southern referred to the Prince Albert, Queen Victoria's husband, the Prince Consort. The portrait had been hung there when the hospital had been built and now it was regarded with affection by everyone working there. The student doctors often adorned the Prince with a bushy beard to go with his mutton-chop whiskers but it was done in the best of humour and no-one would have dreamed of really damaging him, because he was an integral part of the place. He gazed benignly down the length of the hall, watching the comings and goings of the doctors, nurses, patients and visitors, and for a while I gazed absent-mindedly back at him.

I was recalled to my immediate surroundings by a voice addressing us and our names were ticked off against the list. The shortish woman with the dignified manner who stood before us was wearing a dark blue dress. This signified that she was a sister, I recalled from my enquiries at the nursing outfitters. I was immediately proved correct when the speaker introduced herself as home sister, who had come to take us to the Nurses' Home.

"Would you please follow me now," sister added, in a voice that was kindly but brisk. When she started off along the side corridor directly on the left she stepped out briskly too, so that we had to quickly gather up our things and hurry after her. She led us past the kitchens (which we could see and smell), past matron's office (which we did not notice as we trotted by) and then through a door out of the hospital entirely. As we scurried along behind her, I saw that we were now in fact passing over a bridge which spanned the roadway beneath.

This glassed-in covered way was the only access into and out of the Nurses' Home. The home was an entirely separate building from the hospital and was surrounded by a paved area, the lower, basement rooms having windows facing on to this sunken enclosure as many town houses do. The difference was that there were no outside steps down to these rooms. The nurses were defended by a most effective 'moat' with the 'drawbridge' being the covered bridge. It certainly kept the nurses in, and men out (except doctors and porters on official business), but it would have been a terrible fire-risk if there had ever been a fire.

We reached the end of this walkway; the door to the Nurses' Home stood open and we were swiftly shepherded inside, taken along the dark painted corridors and allocated to our individual rooms.

Narrow with high ceilings, painted dark brown like the corridors, the rooms were all equipped with the same things – a high iron bedstead, a single wardrobe, a wash-hand stand with jug and basin, tooth mug and soap dish, and radiator.

I had been allotted one of the basement rooms with less light from the window than those higher up, so it seemed very dark to me as I changed into my uniform and hung my other clothes in the wardrobe. Not a very comfortable room, I thought, but it had all the essentials. It was a little short on luxuries, that was all.

Home sister collected us all together again once we were in our uniforms and took us to one of the lecture rooms to demonstrate to us how to put on our caps. No hair must be showing under the cap and pins or clips were not allowed. This made it all rather more difficult than it first appeared but after a great deal of pulling and tugging and tucking in of stray hair, we passed inspection. Looking at my companions, I supposed I must look as odd as they did, with my own mid-brown short bobbed hair out of sight beneath the stiff white cap. They certainly looked a little strange because in order to cover all the hair at the forehead and temples the caps had to be pulled quite far down. Home sister approved of them, however, and this was all that mattered at the time. I felt that the presence of these caps and uniforms gave definition to the wearers.

We were to discover that as a nurse progressed through her training, the cap crept further back on the head until quite a bit of hair was in fact visible. This was tolerated as long as the whole effect remained clean and tidy, but any straggling wisps of hair were soon noticed and the nurse in question was told to smarten herself up at once.

The uniform was also checked over by home sister at this time. She explained that a neat, clean appearance was the first step along the road to becoming a nurse; the first step and one of the most important to maintain at all times. This was why we must keep our shoes well polished, our hair tidied away, our nails clean, and our dresses and aprons clean. When the aprons, of necessity, got dirty by the nature of our work, we must be changed as soon as practicable – hence the twelve aprons that had seemed to be so many when I was packing them at home would in fact be hardly sufficient for our needs.

We were shown how to fasten our aprons at the back and at the bib with safety pins. The sisters tied their aprons with long white strings, but perhaps because of the extra work involved in ironing such ribbons the junior nurses did not have these, nor did they have bows tied under the chin which made the sisters' caps look so smart.

The separate cuffs were pushed on over our hands. A nurse's cuffs, we were told, could be removed for working but must be replaced when reporting to sister, during doctors' visits, visiting time, or indeed whenever they would not be dirtied.

This need to replace cuffs led to many a hurried hunt around the ward because each nurse grabbed up the nearest pair of cuffs she could find. Sometimes, the last nurse on the ward to look for a pair could not locate them. They might have been left in the ward kitchen, or anywhere around the ward. 'Hunt the cuffs' was a game every nurse soon learned to play.

Home sister then explained to us how to put on the detachable collars in the same way as we might have seen our fathers fasten theirs. As soon as the collars were on, every one of us knew that they were going to rub our necks. The collars were stiff and unyielding – each time we turned our heads, the edge chafed against our skin, rubbing us raw in no time at all. It was a mark of a nurse out of uniform to show a red, sore line around her neck. Luckily, we were soon told by the older nurses that a bar of soap rubbed along the sharp crease of the collar would lubricate it and soften the effect somewhat for us.

Once the home sister had ensured that all the new nurses were acceptable to her, she told us to follow her again. Now that we were all dressed alike in our uniform of purple checks, white aprons, caps and cuffs, black stockings and shoes, we all looked very similar, especially with our hair tucked into our caps. We bore a marked resemblance to a group of chicks scurrying along after their mother hen as we hurried after sister, keen to keep her in view because the last thing she had said to us was 'teatime'.

True to her word, she took us back along the corridors, over the bridge and into the refectory, the nurses' dining hall. Here we saw a great many more nurses all in one place than we had ever seen before, all sitting at long tables with white clothes, with plates and knives in front of each place. The top table was placed at right-angles to the others across the hall, and the sister in charge sat there with the nurses seated in descending order of seniority as we were placed further away from the top table. Home sister ushered us in, showed us where to sit at the bottom of the lowest tables, and then went to the top table to take her place there.

The nurses had all been waiting to begin and now that home sister was there, she said grace and then the food could be passed around. At first, the newcomers waited quietly, watching the big loaves of bread being handed on their platters from one nurse to the next. There was a very blunt bread knife which was handed on as well and each nurse cut herself a large chunk of bread. They could do no better with such a knife. The only butter to be seen was one square in a dish for each table. By the time the bread reached the new probationers at the bottom of the room there was none of this butter left at all. What were we to do? It seemed that we would have to eat dry bread.

There was at least a large teapot on the table so I helped myself to a cup of tea to try to wash the bread down. As I was doing so a nurse a little further up passed a pot of mustard to me and said "Try it with mustard, it helps a bit, you know."

Being a member of a lively family, I suspected a practical joke at first but our new-found friend smiled at us and showed us her own slice of bread smeared thinly with deep yellow mustard. I shrugged, and, raising to my mouth, took a big bite. With a shudder, they watched me chew and swallow the strange mouthful then looked at each other again to see if either one of them dared to follow my example. Perhaps a small smear might be all right. They tried it. It was horrible, but it did help the bread to go down. After a few more teatimes of this sort, we soon began to find nothing odd about eating our bread with mustard.

The reason for this startling diet was simply that the hospital was run entirely by voluntary donations which meant that the staff had to be very mean with their funds. The food was the most basic diet to fill the stomach, and bread and potatoes were high on the list of cheap but bulky food offered to us. Butter was expensive, margarine was not widely known, and jam was a luxury certainly not to be found on the nurses table. If some had been sent from home, it was hoarded along with any cake, biscuits or sweets, all of which the sweet-toothed girls yearned for from time to time, especially when hunger really gripped them in the hours between meals.

The minimal nature of the food was something that they would find out about soon enough, but for now at their first meal on their first day, the new probationer nurses were simply bemused by it all. They struggled to eat their bread, they drank their cups of tea, they gazed about them at the many other nurses there – and they noticed that the new girl who had told them she had already worked for a year at the Eye Hospital was sitting further up the table than the rest of them. It came to them suddenly that this was why the girl had insisted on telling them in the hall that she had already done some training. Seniority had its rewards, one of which was to get a little nearer the top of the table and to stand more of a chance at some of the butter, or anything else that might be passed down.

Sisters ate separately, except those that were on duty in the refectory, so they did not normally participate in this sort of thing, but for the third year probationers, or the senior nurses who had finished their training, the advantage of being at the top was clear. There was always something for those at the bottom, but not always the nicer things, and not always enough.

We rose from the tea table, full but not satisfied, at the summons of home sister once again. All six of us started off after her but one by one she dropped us off at the various wards where we were to start our training. I was taken to the female medical ward and home sister took me in to introduce me to the sister in charge.

We approached the table where the ward sister was writing. She looked up at the two of us and smiled warmly. "Ah, Nurse Knowles" she said. I turned around to look for the nurse that ward sister was addressing, then I turned back to the table in surprise. "It is Nurse Knowles, isn't it?" enquired ward sister, looking at me quizzically. As I nodded in agreement, I realised that the ward sister was addressing me – I was Nurse Knowles – and Nurse Knowles I was now to be for the next three years.

Women's Ward

When I looked around again, I saw that the home sister had left to deliver the rest of her charges to their respective wards and a staff nurse had taken her place. "Come with me," the staff nurse said and took me over to a bed surrounded by screens where a woman lay quietly, very ill and unable to move herself about. She had ascites due to heart failure, commonly called dropsy. "I have prepared this lady for a bed bath. I want you to wash her very thoroughly," said the staff nurse, "and I will come back to help you turn her over once you have done her front."

The woman had been prepared with a waterproof sheet and two blankets, one under and one over her. I washed her carefully with the soap, cloth and basin of warm water provided. I could see that the woman had ascites, a swollen abdomen which was caused by her illness, and made her rather heavy to handle. When I had finished rinsing and drying the patient, the staff nurse came back and asked me if I had washed the umbilicus. "Yes," I replied, because although I didn't yet know that the umbilicus was the medical name for the bellybutton, I did know I had washed the woman's front all over, thoroughly, so I must have washed it whatever it was.

After the staff nurse had shown me how the two of us should turn the patient over, I washed the woman's back. Then we removed the waterproof sheet and blanket by rolling them up, turning the patient on her side and easing her over the roll and removing the sheet and blanket at the other side.

Already I had learnt two or three useful techniques in my first simple task: how to bath a bedridden patient, how to change the bedding while the occupant was still in the bed and, perhaps most importantly, how to move a heavy body without the risk of hurting oneself. "Always use two nurses to move a patient," said the staff nurse as she stood at the other side of the bed, "and always lift together. Ready, Nurse, bend your knees, now – lift!" (Despite all such instructions to new nurses, though, throughout the years a good many nurses have strained their backs and slipped discs through lifting heavy patients, and sometimes found themselves unable to continue their careers because of it).

This particular patient had been too ill to show much response to her bed bath but later on as I worked on the wards I was to find that many people really appreciated them. Patients less ill than the lady I had just bathed, but not well enough to be taken to the ward bathroom, would often enjoy the opportunity of dabbling their hands and feet in a bowl of water while they were being washed.

For the time being, it was enough to absorb the facts, as staff nurse and I put the sheet and blanket away. The bed baths were administered twice a week to patients, their nails were trimmed and cleaned as well, and their hair was washed fortnightly and also just before they went home. It was all part of nursing – to tend and care for the patients' comfort and well-being.

The sister on the female medical ward was in the great nursing mould of Florence Nightingale who had been alive not twenty years before. Sister was a real lady, as kind as could be to nurses and patients alike. She kept very strictly to 'the three Ds' – dedication, discipline, and dignity. I could not have had a better model before me on my first ward.

In the past, the ward sisters had actually lived in little rooms right next to the wards, but now they used each room only as an office whilst they were on duty; writing up notes and discussing patients in there, with the staff nurse or one of the doctors. Each morning for the daily briefing with the ward doctor, the staff nurse would take in a tray of tea and toast for them. Oh, how the sight of that hot buttered toast made me long for a piece for myself.

Matron too had her office, in the corridor to the left of the main entrance hall of the hospital. Unfortunately, it was known to the younger nurses mainly as the place they were summoned to if we had done anything wrong. Also any nurse who had broken a thermometer, or been in attendance when a patient broke one (which was also considered to be the nurse's responsibility), had to go to matron's office to get a replacement. Many nurses preferred to go out and buy one at a cost of 1/6d to themselves rather than turn up in the matron's room to get one free. If, however, as sometimes happened, a whole rack of six thermometers was knocked over or sent flying, there was nothing else to do but to go and see matron, because an outlay of nine shillings was too large an amount out of a nurse's pay all at once.

The salary was not a big consideration to a girl when she decided to become a nurse. If it had been, she would certainly not have taken up that career. The attitude of the hospital was that girls were being trained for a profession, and they were being given their accommodation and meals and part of their uniform, plus washing and cleaning of uniform and room. To pay her as well was really very generous indeed.

This would perhaps not have mattered so much if such things as broken thermometers had not come up occasionally, or indeed the cost of getting home sometimes. Little luxuries like talcum powder and soap also used up some of the £15 which the first year probationers received as their annual pay. I was fortunate because my parents were able to buy my books for me and pay the examination fees.

Even with the small amount they were given, however, the nurses found they were able to afford things, most of their other expenses being met by the hospital and most of their time being spent working or studying, leaving very little time to fritter away their pennies, even if they had had the desire to do so.

They were soon to find out about the long hours; twelve and a half hours a day (or night), with an hour off for dinner and tea. The work was physical; walking, lifting, carrying. It was just as well that almost all the probationers were young, about eighteen years old mostly, because they needed to be fit and healthy to get through the days. (Older women did sometimes train, but married women found it almost impossible because they had to live in whilst they were training and no husband would countenance such a separation for three years without a break).

Even after just an hour or so on the ward, I felt very tired. I had left home, made a journey and begun my career all in one day, so it was no wonder that by the time I left the ward that evening I was ready for some respite. My head was full of new ideas, I was already absorbing some of the basic ways of behaving like a nurse – to look calm and not to panic; to appear cheerful and not to raise my voice; to walk and not to run (except for a fire or a haemorrhage).

When I came off duty at 8.30 p.m. with the other day staff I made my way back to the home for supper. On the way I found out that there was a daily service in the lovely hospital chapel for nurses coming off duty to attend if they wished. So I was refreshed in both mind and body an hour later after a fifteen minute service and a supper of soup. (It was always soup or rice pudding for supper because the cooks had finished for the day and it was simply left out for us to help ourselves).

I spent a little time getting to know people in the sitting room in the Nurses' Home and then wearily made my way to my bedroom. It had been one of the longest days of my life so far, but I felt content as I settled down to sleep. I was here now and my nursing training had well begun. Over the coming weeks on the female ward, I may have lost sight of that feeling of contentment many times but never for too long. I knew I was doing what I wanted to do. Even the food failed to persuade me otherwise.

Breakfast at 7.45 a.m. on my second day was, like the tea of the day before, a very plain affair. We might be served any one of a variety of things, and one was the correct number by which to describe it – one apple, one egg, one slice of bacon, one sardine, or one plate of porridge. The porridge at least was filling and there was always bread.

After some time on this diet, with bread and potatoes as the main constituent, I noticed that although I was working very hard, on my feet all day, and I never felt as though I had enough to eat, I was getting plumper. This was quite clear because my apron wouldn't do up so tightly as the days went on. It was the high carbohydrate intake in the food which was causing it – most of the nurses noticed the same thing. It was hard to believe, but we were putting on weight.

On this, my first full day on the ward, however, I was too full of the newness of things to feel hungry. When I reported to the ward, ready to begin my nursing again, I was surprised when I found myself handed a duster and told to join the others in a flurry of housewife activity.

As I began to polish beside one of the older probationers I was told that matron on her ward rounds, which took place once a week, had an eagle eye for cleanliness on the ward and would seek out any dirt or dust left anywhere around – behind taps in the bathroom, along the picture rail or skirting board – she knew where to look because of course she had been a lowly probationer once upon a time herself and knew all about the high and low dusting which had to be done to keep the wards free from dirt and therefore free from infection.

So every morning, after the night nurse had reported to the day sister and gone off duty at 8.30 a.m., the probationers began their day by going over every surface with dusters and cloths. The ward maid had already cleaned out the two big fire grates, one at either end of the ward, relaid the fires and lit them (unless the weather was warm) and mopped and polished the floor.

These ward maids were often the longest-serving of the ward staff and they were invaluable to the sister, serving as her eyes and ears around the place to tell her of anything amiss while she, perhaps, was not there herself. They could be very helpful and kind to the young nurses but they were each proud of their own ward and wouldn't let any slackness or carelessness let the standard of the ward down.

The maid on the female ward had a habit of putting newspapers down after she had mopped the kitchen floor and this puzzled me quite a bit. If the idea was to keep the floor clean, then why put down papers which marked the floor with newsprint? Of course, I didn't voice my opinion, but I did wonder about it as I went about my own cleaning jobs allocated to me as the most junior probationer, one of which was to polish the chairs, legs, runners, backs and all, ready for the next event of the day – the doctor's rounds.

Before this event, however, I was pleased to discover that we were allowed a tea break after we had cleaned the ward. This twenty minutes was to allow us to wash and tidy ourselves up after the daily cleaning. In that time we had to go back to the Nurses' Home, spruce ourselves up, have a cup of tea and get back to the ward. A bit rushed, to put it mildly, but the tea tasted wonderful and settled the dust in my throat from all the dusting and polishing around the ward which preceded it.

Coming back from the Nurses' Home after the break, washed, hair combed, shoes brushed, clean apron on, I was now ready for the doctor, along with the other nurses, and the ward itself. There was always a doctor's round of some sort, either the junior ward doctor or one of the consultants.

The 'female' was quiet as usual on one such occasion so the doctor's voice sounded quite clearly from behind the screens around one of the beds. No-one was deliberately listening to the conversation but the patients were all in awe of the doctors and especially so during the morning round when they might find out what was to happen to them – whether they were to be allowed home, or to have an operation; so they were always very subdued and the doctor's voice carried well as he encouraged the woman behind the screens.

"Take hold of my hands," he was saying, "hold me tightly now, and pull me towards you as hard as you can."

He was testing the patient's strength and grip, of course, but the other ladies in the ward hearing just the disembodied voice, decided to relieve the tension of the moment by taking quite a different view of it all. They looked at each other and smiled, then one giggled, then another, until that end of the ward was quite merry. No wonder doctors never examined female patients without a nurse in attendance.

I was called upon to attend the doctors while another woman, an Asian lady, received a visit from the student doctors. This woman was causing quite a stir on the ward because she was beautifully tattooed over most of her back. From a line around her neck and wrists the lady was a mass of flowers and animals with a large crucifixion scene in pride of place. She was quite an art gallery but although it was her illustrated body that was causing all the attention, she was actually in hospital for treatment for anaemia.

Part of this treatment was a lot of raw liver in her diet. I was shown how to prepare this in the ward kitchen. It had to be scraped into a sort of paste and made into sandwiches but no matter how I tried to make them look appetising by cutting them up and arranging them on a plate, I knew exactly how the poor woman felt every time I saw her screw her face up at the sight of them, but they seemed to work.

Other medicines and tablets could be unpleasant to take too and they were not always sugar coated either. Some days later, I thought that was why one woman was hesitating before taking her pills. While I was pouring out a glass of water for her to help wash them down, however, the woman asked me very solemnly, "How do these three things know which way to go?" She had been contemplating the pills as they lay in her hand and wondering how the different coloured tablets for her heart, her head and her stomach could possibly know where to travel to once they got down inside her. Her body, as far as she knew, was a solid object, a block with no special pathways to follow and the pills could end up in the wrong places for all she could tell. She was interested but still a bit sceptical to hear it explained that they all went the same way at first but then were absorbed and distributed through the blood to where they were needed. I might know this for a fact from diagrams and lectures, but the patient was less than convinced. It didn't sound nearly as neat and tidy as the woman had always imagined herself to be. Perhaps she didn't like the idea. Still, she swallowed the pills and left the wonders of science to sort it out for themselves after that.

When the time came round for my first day off, I excitedly made the journey home to Fleetwood. I had to go through quite a ritual to get there – waiting at dinner-time the previous day to stand up and ask:

"Sister, it's my day off tomorrow, may I have a late pass and sleep out?"

With this permission at 7 p.m. the next day when I was off-duty I took the train home to Fleetwood to see my parents.

They had so many questions for me and I for them, there was so much to hear about and tell each other, that I had hardly arrived before I found myself coming back the next day on the boat train which came down from Fleetwood at 7.30 p.m. This should have left me plenty of time to get back to the hospital for 10.30 p.m. if only the Manx boat which connected with the boat train had not been held up by the tide. The boat had to wait out at Wyre Light for deeper water and the train had to wait for the boat.

When they finally got under away again, I fretted and fretted all the way back until, at Preston Station, I was actually physically sick with worry. When I had recovered a little, I took the opportunity of the wait there at Preston to spend my last pennies on a phone call to sister to try to explain why I was not going to get back in time, but sister didn't believe such a tall story about boats and tides and trains waiting at docksides.

I arrived back, very late and very distressed. Sister simply enquired, "Was the train late, nurse, or did you miss it?" I could have wept and did so.

The following month, I was determined not to repeat my mistake. I was due off duty at 7 p.m. to catch the train home again, but as 6.30 p.m. approached I was told to give a patient a starch enema. I was not overly concerned about it. I had seen my mother make starch at home, I had made starch poultices on the ward to remove scabs from wounds though I had not seen a starch enema administered. I would certainly be able to do this small task and have plenty of time to get the Fleetwood train.

Alas, for my misplaced confidence.

At 7 p.m. I was still struggling with a thick paste that would have been ideal for a poultice but was far too glutinous to go down the funnel into the enema tube and I knew that I was not going to get home that day. Apologising to the patient, I abandoned my first attempt, threw away the starch paste, washed the equipment and made up a fresh, thin solution of starch. This time I was successful, having learnt by my mistake, but of course I had missed my train and therefore my trip home. I learned later that my parents had been quite worried when I did not arrive on the train as promised. It began to seem that I was not meant to get home to Fleetwood without a fuss.

I was the youngest of the three probationers on the female ward and as such was there to help out where needed, to fetch and carry, to assist the others while still learning all the while. The other two probationers were older, second or third year nurses with more experience and each was in charge of one side of the ward, under the overall supervision of the staff nurse and sister. Each of these girls had about fourteen patients to care for (most of the wards being twenty-eight beds) and to account for each time they reported to the ward sister before they went off duty.

It was by watching them that I learnt the procedure when giving your report. After a frantic search for the stiff cuffs which they all took off while working around the ward, the cuffs were put on, the apron was smoothed down, the cape was straightened and then they stood with their arms stiffly at their sides and gave their report clearly and coherently to sister.

Once, when I was carrying two empty enamel bedpans together across a floor made slippery by the maid's constant polishing, I slipped and dropped the bedpans (which I had been told only to carry one at a time) and chipped them. By standing straight and speaking clearly, I really felt that I had acquitted myself well in front of the sister and got a simple 'don't do it again' as a result. Luckily the bedpans were empty.

Nothing could prepare us for our first death on the wards. I had been nursing a young woman, a teenager like myself, and although I knew that the patient was dying it was still a difficult thing to take in when it came. I wondered if by performing a final service for the girl I would be able to accept that she was really no longer alive, so I asked sister if I could help to lay out the body. Sister must have dealt with hundreds of nurses' reactions to death in her time and she knew this was not the answer. She refused the request kindly and explained.

"My dear, you will have many opportunities to do this in the future. I do not think that you should do it now."

She was probably quite correct to shield me from too much contact with death too soon – better for us to see as much of the healing side of the work as possible at first.

At least this first contact with death had been a gradual process for me. A few months later on the female surgical ward, I was admiring the knitting of one of the post-operative patients, standing by the bed as usual because the nurses were not allowed to sit down to chat. The lady was very pleased to have her handiwork noticed and bent down to the bedside locker to fetch out the knitting pattern for me to see. As she did so, an embolism, a bubble in the blood system, must have reached her heart for she simply slumped down as she lay and when I tried to rouse her, she was found to be dead. This was a real shock to me, to see how suddenly a patient could go, even after she was supposed to be on the road to recovery.

It may have been this experience that made me and the other probationers on the ward feel angry when a husband insisted his wife leave the hospital to help him with the children at home. The woman had suffered a stroke and while she was making good progress, the doctors did not think she was ready to return home yet. It seemed unfair to the young nurses that the patient should be taken away from them before she was completely well. Sister advised them not to be upset because over the years she had often noticed that women kept in hospital away from their family would fret and worry far more than if they were allowed to go back home. Perhaps, she said, the wife would be better off, not worse as we might think.

Gradually, taking such sadness with the enjoyment of seeing someone recover and leave the ward smiling and well again, I began to slip into the routine of the ward until after a month or two it seemed as if I had never been anywhere else or done anything else.

This routine was very important to all those in the ward, nurses and patients alike. It kept things going. Everything got done because it had a time and a place to be done. Nothing could be forgotten so there was little rush and no panic. A comfortable, easy calm surrounded the patients and they could get on with getting well. This was part of the skill of nursing.

I felt it too. It was pleasant to know what you were going to be doing in half an hours time, in two days time, in a weeks time; pleasant to get acquainted with your patients. After an operation or an illness, the patients were kept in hospital, sometimes for a week or a fortnight, until they were judged to be fully recovered. I was content to become 'their' nurse in the weeks they were with me. Hungry I might be, tired I certainly was, chafed by the collar and with sore, blistered feet, but I knew I was doing what I wanted – I was learning to be a nurse.

Men's Ward

Some months later, I was walking briskly down a new ward, the male ward. I was checking for a crooked counterpane to straighten, a bed castor needing to be turned in. If one bed was out of line with the others, my side of the ward would be considered untidy, not up to standard. The new probationers soon learnt that they must keep an eye open for such things, and it had become an affront for any of them to see anything out of place along the ward.

I had just been moved on to the male ward that day and although I had been a little nervous at changing from my first ward to another, I was finding that in the little things at least there was really no difference in nursing, whichever ward it might be. A patient was a person in need of care and attention whether man, woman or child, dirty or clean, friendly or uncooperative. That was another part of learning to be a nurse, not being embarrassed, not noticing the bad things, the unpleasant sights and smells.

Most of the smells on the wards were actually nice rather than nasty. In the main, the hospital simply smelt clean, as it should do with all the scrubbing and polishing, sweeping and dusting that the maids and the nurses put into it. One distinctive thing about the separate wards, though, was their individual aroma and disinfectants.

I glanced down at the bed where a patient leaned back against his pillow blowing a cloud or two of smoke from his pipe. The wives never brought flowers to the men, only the strong 'bacca' which the men insisted on for their pipes or hand rolled cigarettes. The female wards smelt of scented talcum powder and flowers but the male wards smelt of tobacco. The man took the pipe from his mouth and smiled up at me. "Nurse, may I have the screens, please?"

"Certainly," I answered, but getting the screens was not as simple as it sounded.

All the new nurses tried to push or pull the screens along on their castors – after all, that was what castors were for – but the top-heavy swaying of the frames, the squealing and grumbling of the wheels, and the way one section of a screen suddenly headed off in a totally different direction, made the screens so difficult to control that they quickly opted to carry them instead.

The reason for the castors jamming, which was what caused the screens to be so awkward, was that although they were cleaned thoroughly each week as part of the ward routine, they never got their castors oiled. The nurses did not carry oil cans in their apron pockets! So, despite the cleaning, the castors still picked up any dirt left on the clean ward floors until one of them locked solid.

I had to carry three of these heavy screens over to the bed and then spread them out to cover both sides and the end of the bed to provide an effective barrier. Then, turning away, I walked back down to the ward, smoothing my big white apron and checking my cap to make sure it was still correctly in place.

The bedside lockers had been cleaned out that morning, lunch had been served and cleared away, and now the patients were quiet for a while, reading the newspapers brought in before lunch by the paperboy, smoking their pipes or cigarettes (which they were allowed to do in the afternoons while the ward windows were open to keep the atmosphere clear), or snuggled down in bed dozing the time away until dinner. A normal, routine day just like many others during my three months on the female ward.

About five minutes later a plaintive voice floated out from behind the screens.

"Nurse, I asked you for the screens please."

"Well," I replied rather puzzled, "you have them." And I carried on down the ward; getting a tin of biscuits out of his locker for another patient who could not reach down to get them himself, folding up and putting away a newspaper that had slipped to the floor as the reader fell asleep.

"Nurse, please, the screens," the disembodied voice called out again. This time it really sounded quite distressed.

Bustling back towards the screens, I noticed the man in the bed next to the screened one was trying to tell me something.

"He means he wants a bedpan, Nurse. We always ask for the screens when we want a bedpan. I just thought I'd explain to you to save his embarrassment, you see."

Save his embarrassment, indeed! If only people would say what they meant. As I hurried to the poor man's relief with a bedpan, I reflected wryly that some things were different on different wards – the men were not quite as straightforward in voicing their requests as the women.

I was not the only probationer with a lot still to learn. A few days later I noticed one of the other new nurses beckoning to me from the doorway of the ward bathroom. Someone was laughing inside the room but the nurse's face was a picture of concern. This was soon explained when I went into the bathroom and saw who was doing the laughing.

It was one of the patients. He had been prescribed a potassium permanganate bath as a treatment for a skin disease. Soaking in a warm bath of any sort was usually very soothing for the patients but in this case the soaking had produced a startling result. The young nurse had only ever seen big handfuls of salt thrown into the water to make a saline bath and the equally large amount of potassium permanganate she had used had turned the water dark purple – and the patient dark brown!

When he got out of the bath both he and the nurse could see that up to the level of the water he was a dark tan colour, above that the usual town-dweller's off-white. It was this half and half effect that he was finding so hilarious; the nurse was not in the least amused. She thought that staff nurse and ward sister would not find it funny either and of course she was quite right.

There was nothing to be done to remove the stain. No treatment mild enough to leave the skin intact was strong enough to shift the colour. It might seem callous, but to the worried probationer the state of the bath was of far more significance than the state of the man. After all, he had no real ill-effects and in time the colour would fade, but the bath was stained brown half way up its sides and liberally splashed with rusting looking marks above that.

The poor girl had to go and report it to staff nurse and then she found herself in front of sister. She was told to spend her free time working on the bath until it was white again. It took her a great many hours to do it and it never really did come up white again.

In the meantime, the man himself was quite a celebrity on the ward, showing the other patients the beautiful colour of his lower self and the exact line at which it stopped. His fun and games were only halted by his wife's reaction when she came to visit him that evening. She didn't enter into the spirit of the thing at all.

It was a scandal, she said, turning her husband into a freak like that, it shouldn't be allowed, something should be done about it. But nothing could be done – as the nurse had found out to her cost – so until nature gradually faded him, he continued to be proud of his tide mark among his mates and sorry for it when his wife came in to see him.

'Learning on the ward' was the main way of teaching nurses at this time accompanied by lectures in the lecture-room of the Nurses' Home. (The only time that men were allowed into the home, apart from the porters, was when the doctors crossed the bridge to give lectures to the nurses). The new nurses learnt by watching and assisting and under supervision they didn't make any serious mistakes. Minor mishaps probably only helped the learning process along. After my episode with the screens, I would always remember that patients didn't necessarily say what they meant and my colleague would never forget the potassium permanganate incident, so perhaps the very occasional little mistake was a good thing, even if – once in a blue moon – it wasn't the probationer that made it.

One morning staff nurse had called everyone to a patient lying on his left side with a green cloth spread across his upper right side from ribs to abdomen. She was explaining the age-old use of leeches to reduce inflammation over the liver area and while the nurses concentrated on her words, no-one was sparing a glance for the six shiny black leeches which were busily sucking away at the patient's skin through small slits made in the green cloth.

Staff nurse had already shown the probationers how to position the leeches using forceps to take them from their laboratory jar and place them on the cloth. Neither nurse nor patient had any contact with them except where they latched on to the patient through slits made in the cloth just over the area to be treated. Now she was describing the beneficial effects of this very ancient form of treatment when she was suddenly interrupted by another patient who had been passing by.

"One of these things has fallen off," he said, attempting to hand her a fat, glistening black shape. "Do you want it back?"

As she told them at the beginning of her talk that they must make certain all leeches went back to the laboratory where they were bred, the staff nurse most assuredly did want it back. She took the thing from him using a piece of gauze and put it back into its jar at once. The other five were still where they should be, attached to the patient in the bed.

This accident was in fact a perfect demonstration of how leeches should not be removed from the skin – that is to say, they should be allowed to drop off one by one as they become too full to hang on any more and, satiated, relax their jaws. They should never be pulled off because while the leech is feeding the mouth parts are locked in the flesh and the leech's saliva containing an anti-clotting agent, hirudin, would be left in the wound to cause further bleeding and infection.

Staff nurse had taken the unexpected opportunity to press home this point to her group but although the probationers nodded to show they were taking the lesson to heart, they all knew it had definitely not been intended to be a part of her lecture.

On a specialist's rounds one memorable day, I was the object of a lecture from the exalted person of the doctor himself.

He had asked for 'a B.P., please' and as the most junior person there I had scampered away to the sluice room and chosen the newest, shiniest, least chipped bedpan I could find there. Covering it with a cloth in the usual way, I hurried back and presented it at the bedside, to the huge amusement of the doctor and students and the suppressed annoyance of sister, who wanted her nurses to be seen as efficient, not laughed at for getting things wrong.

What a grand man that doctor was. Seeing my dreadful embarrassment, he stifled his own mirth, shushed his students and told me I had been quite right as far as my training went to assume he wanted me to bring a bedpan. I could not know yet, he said, of the other two B.P.s he might have meant. Smiling at me, he explained that he had actually wanted a blood pressure apparatus (which was quite an innovation at the time and always administered by the Doctor himself) but he could also have been asking me to bring him a copy of the British Pharmacopoeia, the huge book used by doctors when prescribing, which listed all the drugs.

Now, he said, as another nurse brought the blood pressure apparatus to the bedside, we must all take note of this and remember to make our instructions clear, in case they should be innocently misinterpreted as in this case. Then, while he explained the use of the Blood Pressure apparatus to the students round the bed, I was left to recover from my moment in the spotlight and to reflect as I took the bedpan back to the sluice room that the most senior of people could be the nicest.

Bringing bedpans and bottles, giving bed baths, washing and feeding patients, dusting the ward, changing the beds, still made up most of my work at this stage of my training, and sometimes other, less frequent but still very mundane things. Mundane, but all aimed at making the patients more comfortable and better cared for. That was why one dark winter afternoon found me standing on the ward table, having climbed up via a chair, in the centre of the ward, changing a light bulb before I switched on the lights in the gloom.

I had removed the broken bulb and replaced it with a good one and was just stepping back down when my foot went right through the chair seat and I found myself stuck in a very awkward position.

Most of the patients were dozing at that time of the day but one man had been watching me and saw the accident. He had jumped up from his bed, run over and caught me round the waist before I realised what was happening. He steadied me while I freed my foot and then when I turned to thank him I found myself face to face with the last patient I would have expected to be able to come to my assistance. The man had been shell-shocked since the Great War and supposedly unable to respond. No-one had ever seen him so much as smile at anyone before.

It was found after this that he was able to leave the hospital. He wasn't completely cured, physiotherapy and psychiatry would still be needed but there was one very encouraging sign – he did say he had enjoyed giving a nurse a hug and a squeeze in the interests of saving her from falling.

Some patients in particular needed constant nursing. One man on my side of the ward and therefore under my special care was suffering from cancer of the tongue.

The treatment for this type of cancer was radium. Treatment with radium was still very much in its infancy. At the special Radium Hospital in Liverpool, hollow needles as thick as a fine knitting needle and as long as a darning needle were filled with various doses of radium salt, then closed with screwed tops. The tops had strings threaded with coloured beads (the colour of the beads denoted the strength of the radium).

The needles were delivered from the Radium Hospital in a lead-lined box carried by a long handle to keep it well away from the messenger's body. Then they were inserted into the tumour under a general anaesthetic in the operating theatre. Dosages were carefully calculated to kill off the cancer while harming as little of the surrounding tissue as possible.

Once the patient was back on the ward it was I who checked the needles and made sure they were securely in place with their coloured beaded threads taped firmly to the outside of the cheek. A colleague double-checked, counting the needles as the nurses came on and off duty and we both signed a book stating that everything was correct. If a needle was mislaid around the ward it could have given a dose of radiation to an already sick patient, so the needles were checked and re-checked and used needles were locked away in their lead-lined box to go back to the Radium Hospital.

Each time I cleaned the patient's mouth, I anaesthetised the area with spray. The patient could take a little of his liquid diet while the needles were in place and then his mouth was cleaned again. All of this had to be done within ten minutes to minimise any effects of the radium on me. It was far from pleasant for him or myself.

Naturally, the man had to be coaxed to take any food because of the pain. With regular cleaning and feeding, and trying to prevent his mouth and lips drying out, I did my best to make him feel comfortable while he was confined to bed. After the needles had been removed he was allowed to move about more freely while he completed his time on the ward.

Later, when he could speak without distress, he began talking about his life in a lodging house at the top of Hill Street. There, his life was hard and miserable, while in the hospital all his needs were attended to. He had been in pain but nothing else had been a worry to him and he had obviously appreciated this. I thought I understood why he felt as he did but I did not guess the depth of those feelings. I was completely unprepared when one day, while he was walking about to regain his strength, he came up to me and took my face gently between his hands and asked me to marry him.

My first instinct was to laugh, but looking at him I realised that he was only responding to the care and attention he lacked in the rest of his workload. I could only think it quite natural that he wanted to keep some of that atmosphere through me. Quietly I told him I was dedicating my life to nursing and nurses were not allowed to marry whilst in training. I hoped he would understand and he seemed to accept it, so I felt my refusal hadn't hurt his feelings too much.

A few days later he left the hospital but after each of his weekly clinic visits he came back to the ward bringing with him an apple, or an orange, or a flower for me. I was really touched because these single items represented quite an expenditure for him.

Most of the people treated in the hospital were poor. The rich were mostly nursed at home privately. Chronic cases were sent straight to the municipal hospitals or they were transferred there after diagnosis. This meant that the Royal Southern had a turnover of patients who appreciated the clean beds and regular food and this led to a strange chain of events over Christmas one year.

The doctor on the men's ward naturally assumed that patients would prefer to be at home for Christmas and also that the nurses would prefer a quiet ward over the holiday period, so he very kindly went around the beds giving permission for the discharge of anyone he judged able to go home. It was a shock to him, therefore, to come in on Christmas Day and find all the men still there. He asked sister why she had not discharged the patients he had indicated and she told him most of them would spend a 'more comfortable' Christmas in hospital. They came from the hostels around the docks area of Liverpool and it was not in their best interests to let them go – and she didn't need to mention that they were quite willing to remain. Everyone looked happy and content, clean and neat in their hospital pyjamas between clean sheets with the Christmas decorations up around the ward and the prospect of turkey and plum pudding for dinner, and a visit from Father Christmas.

Nurses, unless they had an infectious illness or a boil or an infected wound, could not stay in bed off duty. Colds, sore feet, headaches, and so on were to be endured while we worked. I was struggling on with a heavy, feverish cold, keeping a smile on my face as I walked along the ward when a man at the far end of the thirty bed ward asked me to get him some more barley water. Head buzzing, limbs aching, I went to his bed to get the empty jug, carried it down to the ward kitchen to fill it and took it back along the ward to him, feeling all the while that I should have been tucked up in bed with barley water of my own. Just as I put the jug down on the locker, the patient in the next bed looked up and said "That looks good, I'll have some too." How I longed for visiting time.

No trips for drinks, no bedpans or bottles during visiting times, no screens to shift, no beds to make, no changing of dressings. I could sit at the ward table instead, making up squares for dressings and stacking them inside the dressing drums ready for sterilisation. When each drum was packed, the porters took them to the sterilising room. Their ventilation holes were opened during this process and then closed while still scalding hot to keep every possible germ at bay. There were always dressings to be made up for the wards and for theatre as well. It was restful work while the visitors were there and I could sit down to do it.

There would be time to relax a little and time to hear a stray remark from the visitors as well, perhaps the 'potassium' man's wife complaining about the colour of her husband which had still not quite faded, or perhaps a little comment that had me struggling to keep a straight face one evening while I folded the gauze.

An elderly man had been admitted for surgery for removal of his prostate gland and was convalescing well after his operation. Prostatectomy was what is said on his records, but his wife chatting to the lady visitor at the next bed didn't get it quite right. According to her, her husband had had his prostitutes removed, and was feeling a lot better for it.

Theatre

Once I had become used to the routine of the wards, I found myself truly enjoying my training, long hours and discomforts notwithstanding. So naturally, as I was beginning to feel comfortable, I was immediately moved on to spend my next few months in the operating theatre.

So far as I knew at the time I was moved, theatre was simply the place patients were wheeled off to, and returned from later to be watched over carefully until they recovered from the anaesthetic. I also knew that patients often didn't wake up feeling as instantly cured and completely well as they had been expecting after their operation, certainly not directly afterwards, anyhow. On the contrary, they usually hurt somewhere or other to a greater or lesser degree from the surgery, and they often felt dizzy and nauseous from the anaesthetic.

This had been particularly well illustrated for me by one particular man who had been very insistent about the fact that he was an atheist when I had been filling in the details on his hospital notes and asked him about his religious denomination. I had been treated to a little lecture on atheism and I knew that the men in the beds round about him had the same treatment and they were all extremely well aware that he was an atheist by the time he was ready to go down to theatre. It was in truth unusual in 1929 not to have any religious belief at all, or at least not to pay lip-service to some denomination or other if nothing else, but this patient was so very proud of the fact that he answered to no gods at all but himself, he made sure everyone knew.

Now, on the day he was to go down to theatre for his surgery he was still an atheist, right up until he was given the anaesthetic he was an atheist, but when he came back to the ward after his operation he was wheeled in on the Theatre trolley and transferred to his ward bed. He was awake from the anaesthetic but he was still somewhat groggy, when everyone in the ward suddenly heard him shout, "Oh, my God!

Oh, my God!   Oh, my God!" over and over again in his semi-conscious state, until I went to attend to him and managed to soothe him into being quiet again.

Poor man! He may not have meant to call on God, probably he just used the most familiar form of words to ease him in his pain, but I knew he would never live it down among the other men on the ward. I had seen him before his operation boring them all with his talk of not believing in God, seen them all wishing that, like Lazarus, they could take up their beds and walk as far away from him as possible so as not to get the lecture on religion and his unbelief.   They had been put through it then, so nothing was more certain from the smiles on their faces than that they would put him through it now and tease him unmercifully without a let-up until the day he was discharged home. And they did.

His reaction under anaesthetic was not an unusual occurrence. Having seen others come back babbling in their sleep from theatre, many a strong man, and many a nervous woman too, worried about how they would behave under the anaesthetic. Would they yell, say something silly or, worse still, something rude? Would they thrash about, hit someone or break something?   If anyone voiced these worries, the nurses always reassured them, but faced with evidence of their ward companions the patients were not always convinced. How things have changed today!

In fact, the nurses knew that some patients would be difficult to deal with once the anaesthetic was being administered. In particular, any heavy beer drinkers among the men were difficult to put under. (This included most of the men; labourers drank a great deal of beer during and after their work to replace body fluid, and down on the dockside the warehouses were interspersed with dockers' pubs every hundred yards or so. It was an accepted way of life).

The patients were usually given atropine to prepare them for the anaesthetic while they were in bed in the ward about half an hour before the operation was to take place.   After they had been transferred to the trolley and wheeled along to theatre, they were anaesthetised before being taken through into the theatre proper. The anaesthetist administered chloroform mixed with ether by dripping it on to a mask placed over the patient's mouth and nose. This was done in the anteroom to the operating theatre after the final checks for the operation.

It was at this point that a big, beer-drinking man would really cause problems if not dealt with properly because he would take a lot of anaesthetic for it to have the desired effect. His body, accustomed to drugs from frequently drinking large amounts of alcohol, took longer to absorb the anaesthetic than might have been judged from body weight alone, and as he found himself slipping slowly away the man would try to fight the effects as he went under. Going under the effect of ether and chloroform was frightening – not like modern anaesthetics which are quick and easy.

The anaesthetist, by asking questions and from long experience, could usually tell which of his patients were likely to be difficult and if he thought they were going to give trouble he would have them strapped across the chest and around the knees to hold them firmly on the trolley, because otherwise as their arms and legs jerked and banged around they might damage themselves, or hurt a nurse or doctor, or smash equipment, until they quietened down and were completely unconscious at last.

(Some years later, when I myself had an anaesthetic for a small operation, I found out what it was that patients experienced when I had to undergo it in my turn. The effect, I felt, was like spiralling up and up into the sky, somewhat like the scene in the Wizard of Oz when the house is picked up by a tornado and taken round and round, higher and higher, faster and faster, until – nothing! Nothing, that is, until the wakening back in the ward. A horrible, whirling, sickening feeling. No wonder the men fought against it).

One teenage girl who had apparently become pregnant but whose blood tests were negative was due to be taken into theatre for an examination of her swollen abdomen. As soon as she was unconscious under the anaesthetic the swelling subsided and the abdomen became flat. The patient returned to the ward, where she swelled up again once she regained consciousness. This strange case was in fact a phantom pregnancy which the girl had brought about herself. She came from a very strict family and when she allowed her boyfriend to kiss her she became convinced that she would have a baby because she had been 'bad'. It took many sessions with the psychiatrist to show her not only that pregnancy did not occur in this way, but that she had done nothing wrong at all and should stop punishing herself.

General anaesthetics were only used for major surgery. As with any anaesthetic there is always a risk of an adverse reaction or problems of one sort or another. Minor operations and some internal examinations were done in the theatre but under a local anaesthetic, an injection into the area to be operated upon or examined. This was a less traumatic, simpler way of dealing with these small theatre visits.

Cystoscopies (examinations of the bladder) were performed in this way, when a tube was passed up into the bladder to enable the surgeon to look right inside and check for any inflammation or abnormality. It was quite a common procedure, often three or four would be done in a morning, following each other quite quickly into theatre. Cystoscopy, although it was one of the many new and unusual words that I had to remember, was one which I knew I would never forget after my first experience with it.

Long before being moved to work in theatre, indeed while I was still on the female ward and very new to nursing, staff nurse had called me over to one of the windows which overlooked the hospital grounds and pointed out a doctor playing tennis on one of the grass courts below them.

"Nurse," she said, "Go down and tell Dr Papvovski that his cystoscopies are ready for him to see now," and she sent me on my way.

All along the corridors, down through the hospital and out into the gardens, I rehearsed and rehearsed my little speech until I stood at the side of the court, caught the doctor's attention and announced, "Mr Cystoscopy, your papvovskies are ready."

Luckily, Dr Papvovski, although foreign, understood a slip of the tongue when he heard it and he had a strong sense of humour and took it very well, but I still winced for my own discomfiture whenever I recalled my mistake. And I tended to recall it every time I attended a cystoscopy in theatre, which was fairly frequent day by day. I was remembering it now, on this particular day, while I stood by the head of yet another lady undergoing the self-same examination.

I was there to reassure and keep watch over the patient while behind a large green-draped screen the surgeon was studying the inside of the woman's bladder through a cystoscope. Unusually for this most routine of procedures, however, the patient seemed to be suffering some distress, screwing her mouth up and pulling faces until finally she let out a small moan. I bent down at once to ask her if she was all right. I received no answer to my enquiry, but a little later the woman moaned again. Again I bent towards her and asked "Are you all right, my dear?" and again there was no answer. When the woman groaned a third time, the surgeon decided to pop his head around the screen.

Knowing she could definitely not be in any actual pain because of the local anaesthetic she had been given, and thinking she must simply be embarrassed at her undignified position while the examination was being carried out, he told her cheerfully not to worry, they had seen plenty of bladders before! Her answer struck him dumb, along with the rest of the theatre staff.

"Oh, I'm not worried about that," she mumbled dismissively, "but, dear oh dear, I haven't got my teeth in!" Vanity, vanity!

The real problem with being in theatre was that there were very few light moments of that sort, hardly any contact with the patients at all. I never felt at home there. People weren't in need of friendly care and attention, they were just draped shapes on the table to be dealt with; everything had to be done quickly and efficiently and without emotion, like a machine-shop, to my mind, everything had to be scrubbed and sterilised, everything had to be precisely in its place. There was no room for a human being at all! Added to this, I found that my glasses steamed up above my mask in the hot, humid atmosphere and this restricted vision made me slow and awkward until I learned the trick of polishing the lenses with soap before I went into theatre, but by this time I had already drawn the unfavourable attention of theatre sister, who was most efficient.

Sadly too, when it came to my first attendance at an amputation, I found I knew the patient who was to undergo the operation. A pleasant lady that I had nursed on the ward had developed gangrene in her leg. As so often happened, amputation became the only way of saving a life once gangrene had deeply affected the limb. Everyone knew it was the best, the only, treatment but it was never a pleasant thing to have to do although it was still quite common. Every nurse had to go through it, like their first death on the ward, but I wished it could have been someone I didn't recognise.

I had to think hard about the alternative, death, for this patient if she did not have her leg removed before I managed to subdue my feelings and regain a degree of calm which I badly needed at that time. Above all, I reminded myself, I must not faint. Theatre sister would be sure to make a great fuss about me being 'unsuitable' if I did because I was already in her bad books; it was usually important to remain calm and in control as I knew allowances would not be made for me. I had armed myself with all my colleagues' recollections of their first time assisting in this operation, so I kept my mind well away from the draped figure on the table and when I was asked to hold the leg, I did so stoically throughout the cutting and sawing, keeping my eyes to the front and not to the side where the surgeon was working away. Only when I felt the leg come away in my hands did all my mental preparation go for nothing.

I didn't faint but for a moment I could only stand in shock and wonder what on earth to do with the leg. Should I take the leg away now, right out of the theatre; should I hand it to someone else to deal with, or what? I looked over at theatre sister in desperation and sister indicated with a flicker of her eyes that there was a bucket beside me to put the leg into. I moved to the bucket but then stood still again wondering, which way up I should place the leg in the bucket? Should it be foot first because if I turned the leg up the other way the blood would flow out from the seared end; or amputation site first, to keep the bloody end of the leg away from the sterile gowns and drapes. It felt like the beginning of a nightmare, holding the leg in my hands, unable to make up my mind. Well, there was no time to hesitate, sister was looking round in annoyance. She took a deep breath and said, "put the leg in the bucket foot upwards" and I raised my eyes to look at sister again. A tight smile told me I had got it right.

I might have passed that test but even so I found throughout my weeks there I could not please theatre sister. It wasn't surprising really because no matter how I tried I couldn't make myself enjoy theatre work. I couldn't take what seemed to me to be the dehumanising aspect of it. So of course it was natural that theatre sister was less than pleased with me, which completed my discomfiture. Sister noticed every one of my mistakes and told me about them, whilst letting other nurses get by without a reprimand, as often as not, or so it began to seem to me.

Perhaps that was why one morning theatre sister found when she put her feet into her white theatre boots that someone had filled them with cold water beforehand. Maybe that someone was trying to inject some fun into the deadly serious theatre atmosphere, or maybe she just wanted to make life a little difficult for someone who had made her life really hard. At any rate, sister never found out who did it and none of the other nurses, laughing behind their serious faces, ever told her that I had finally had my revenge.

No-one would have dreamed of giving another nurse away over a little practical joke like that, a united front was always shown in such cases. The atmosphere in the Nurses' Home was something like a boarding school, everyone stuck together.

After their long hours on duty, the nurses would hurry back to the Nurses' Home to gather in the sitting room and relax and chat. If I arrived before the sofa was taken, I could sit across the cushions with my legs up on the arm to give my poor, aching feet a rest after my twelve hour day and let the blood drain back out of my swollen ankles. If I was late, others would have taken the favoured positions and I, like all the rest, had to make do with the four or five easy chairs, or the floor if I had to. In their sitting room the girls could let themselves go, sisters and staff nurses had their own sitting rooms, so no-one disturbed them. The fire in the hearth, the end of work for the day, the companionship of the other nurses, were all their own for a while. I loved the chattering, friendly atmosphere; coming from a family of four sisters it felt quite homely and I slipped easily into the routine of the place.

Feet were becoming a very important subject to everyone in the Nurses' Home; resting them, bathing them, keeping swelling at bay were major occupations and topics of conversation for the nurses in these evening gatherings. Someone once took a pedometer round with her strapped to her ankle just out of interest to see how far she walked in one day on the wards. The little wheel clocked up twelve miles during a fairly ordinary days work.

After resting in the sitting room, feet up on the sofa arm if possible, a foot bath was often a quick way to revive, if a whole body soak in a really deep hot bath itself was out of the question, through tiredness or queues for the bathroom. As often as not the sitting room was littered with enamel bowls, full of hot water and bare feet, while their owners discussed a patient, or sister, or when they were next due to go home, above the Epsom salts or saline, whichever was the preferred soaking solution for that particular nurse and the cheapest.

But a proper, deep, hot bath was the real life-saver for me and for anyone else who could arrange one. The bathrooms in the home were constantly in use during the evenings, one nurse sometimes running a fresh bath while she was towelling herself dry, to speed things up for the next occupant of the bathroom and help give more girls a chance to really unwind from the tensions of the day, unknotting tired muscles and easing aching backs.

One nurse had started a bath running for a friend and left it running as she went back to her own room, pausing as she went along the corridor to knock on her friend's door to let her know the bathroom was ready for her. Unfortunately, her friend had given up the idea of ever getting to the bathroom that night and had gone to have a chinwag in the sitting room instead with the other nurses. The water kept running, the plug was firmly in the plug hole, no-one else came to see if the bathroom was free for quite a while – but when they did they were in good time to see the water pouring over the side of the bath like a miniature Niagara, all over the floor, round the edges of the linoleum and down through the cracks in the floorboards to splash and splatter through the ceiling of the corridor beneath and form great puddles all along the passageway downstairs.

Cries for help from the nurse in the bathroom as she quickly turned off the taps and pulled out the plug to stop the continuing waterfall were coupled with more distant shrieks and squeals from the corridor downstairs as the girls came out of their rooms to investigate the strange noise of bath-water dripping like rain through their ceiling. More and more of the nurses were drawn out of their rooms by the growing uproar to stand and gaze aghast at the scene of devastation.

Everyone simply stood there amazed for a minute or two, until they realised what was happening. After a moment, people began to rush up and down the stairs to see the other half of the problem and then, realising what had to be done, they all set to with mops and buckets to clear up the mess.

Next morning all was back to normal, – only the maid who cleaned and polished in the Home was suspicious, when she noticed that all the shine was off her floors in the ground floor corridor that day, but not one of the nurses seemed to know anything about it.

Statistically, there were a lot of mishaps involving baths in the Nurses' Home. Perhaps this was because everyone took a daily bath and that added up to a lot of bath water each day. Baths frequently splashed over and soaked the lino floor making the next occupant complain that there was nowhere to dry to put her clothes, and often a nurse would spend far too long indulgently soaking herself, making other people wait, which they of course thought most unfair but learned to accept philosophically. After all, they in their turn might overstay their own time given the opportunity.

One evening, however, a small crowd had gathered outside the bathroom, looking worried. It seemed to me, next in line to use the bathroom, that I had been waiting such a long time, so I hammered quite loudly on the door and asked how long I was expected to wait. I was first angry and then alarmed when I got no answer to my knocking, so I had fetched a chair from my room and managed to peer in through the fanlight above the door just enough to catch a sight of the bath itself. What I saw frightened me and sent me off to get home sister's help. The bath water was stained red and the girl in the bath was slumped right down in the water, head back on the rim of the bath, lolling on one side. The crowd now awaited my return with sister to find out what had happened.

Home sister had a master key to all the rooms in the Nurses' Home and when she bustled up with the anxious nurse it was very simple for her to unlock the door from the outside and step into the bathroom to discover – a nurse fast asleep in a warm, soothing bath and a red coloured binding on a book which was floating in the water where it had slipped from her hand as she dropped off to sleep. The colour was the only thing that had 'bled' into the bath. The nurse awoke to a room full of gawping girls and a sister who was not amused at having been called from her quiet evening to attend a non-existent emergency. It was a novel as well, not even a reference book.

For a while after this incident the nurses were careful to be in and out of the bathroom quickly, and as a consequence quite a few more nurses were able to get a bath each evening for a few weeks while the memory of the sleeping bather was fresh in their minds. It was my luck to be the last in a long line in the bathroom one night. I had taken advantage of being last to enjoy the luxury of a good soak in peace and quiet and had been thoroughly enjoying myself when, as I was drying myself off after the water had finished gurgling away down the plug hole, I began to get the feeling that perhaps it was a little bit too quiet.

It was very late I knew and it seemed that all the other nurses had decided to settle down for the night and had already gone to bed, for I found I couldn't hear anyone through the bathroom door. As I dressed myself in my warm night things and tidily straightened things up around the room, I kept listening out until the silence became almost uncanny. I was straining my ears, listening for a cheerful 'goodnight' or voices talking low in one of the bedrooms as friends gossiped on into the night, but there was nothing at all. The other little night-time noises, floorboards creaking, wind rustling outside, were heightened against the lack of human sound. It was rather eerie. I found myself reluctant to go out into the darkened corridor from the bright, warm bathroom.

Still, finally gathering up my towel and soap, I told myself briskly not be silly and opened the door. As I did so the draught from the cold passageway rushed into the steamy room and must have caught the window blind behind me where it hung down over the bathroom window. The sudden gust of wind sent the blind flapping and whirring its way back up on to its roller making quite the loudest noise I thought I had ever heard. I didn't wait to reason out what had happened at the time though, I just rocketed off down the corridor as fast as I could go, flew into my own room, slammed the door and leaned against it breathing heavily, all the hairs on the back of my neck standing up on end.

After I had scrambled into bed, I had to then get out to put the light out, then shot back under the covers again, and I worked out what must have caused it all. I stopped shivering as I calmed down and warmed up in bed and was just thinking that after such a fright I would never be able to get to sleep, when I woke next morning to the maid's call at 7 a.m. – "Nurse!"

It was like that every night, neither I nor any other of the nurses had any time left at the end of the day to feel afraid, or worry too much about things, or to get neurotic; we worked too hard and were left feeling too tired for luxuries like that.

Children's Ward

What a contrast came next for me. The sister on the children's ward was so different from theatre sister. At first she seemed rather laughable, sitting on the end of a child's bed singing 'Jesus wants me for a sunbeam' with her short legs swinging in time to the music an inch or two above the floor, but her sweet Welsh singing voice was nearer to her true nature. Inside she was all sunshine and love for the children in her care.

There was quite a strong Welsh contingent in the Royal Southern Hospital. The orthopaedic surgeon, 'Pinky' Williams, often had patients brought up from Wales for operations, as one lady remarked she had come "all the way from Balla in an ambulance indeed." On the children's ward there were four Nurse Jones' – the only time a nurse was referred to by her Christian name was to differentiate between them – plus, of course, sister herself. From North Wales the nearest large city was Liverpool so naturally Welsh patients, nurses and doctors arrived there in force.

It was a good thing for the children that the nurses on their ward were as loving as they could be, because parents were certainly not allowed to stay with the children while they were in hospital. In fact, there were often no visitors at all for some of the patients – they could too easily spread infection in the ward – in these cases they could only smile and wave to the children through the glass partition.

It made the task of nursing these little ones more exacting to be the only adult available to the child. I found myself in charge of one little girl who had been admitted with an infected ear. An opening had been made behind the ear to allow it to drain but the child had developed infection elsewhere, in the chest or pleural cavity, producing pleurisy and then empyema which also had to be drained. The child was very ill for a time, and her parents came six or seven miles each day to stand at the door and anxiously watch their daughter.

Under careful nursing, the child recovered gradually and over the weeks I got into the habit of telling her a story each evening before she settled down to sleep. Beginning this routine while the girl was still very ill, I continued until the tale was so well known that any slight deviation from the tale caused my listener to protest, "No, no, you're getting it wrong!" The story was one that I knew off by heart myself. It had been told to me many times by my own mother when I was small. I knew plenty of other tales but my patient never wanted to hear any of them. She insisted on the one about the little girl and her dog.

A little girl went with her little dog, Rover, for a walk in the woods. She wandered a long way and then stopped to eat her picnic (but she hadn't packed anything for Rover to eat and she didn't give him any of her food either). Then, when she tried to find the way back home, she discovered she was lost, and as night fell, she was so tired that she lay down to try to sleep on the ground under the tree. Her faithful dog, despite not having any food all day, stayed with her and curled up beside her to guard her and keep her warm. In the morning the little girl realised how Rover had looked after her while she slept and promised the dog a big bone if ever they got home again. Then, with Rover sniffing out the way, they found their way back home and lived happily ever after!

When the little patient was well enough for her parents to visit, they regularly brought cakes for her when they came in the evening. They also brought an extra cake each time for me because they had seen how their daughter's eyes followed me as I moved up and down the ward and they knew she had found someone to rely on while they were unable to be there to help. After the child was discharged from hospital, I still kept in touch and they invited me to visit them at their home. I did go to see them and I remained firm friends with the family for years and I am still in contact with the grown up child.

One mother, though, was not so friendly. Glancing across at visiting time, I seemed to see blood on the woman's hand as she reached to pick up her child from its bed in the ward. Certainly, something must be wrong, the mother's fingers appeared to be bright red. I spoke at once, "Oh, have you cut your finger?" and I received a frosty stare in reply. Putting her infant down again, the woman displayed her red painted nails to my astonished gaze and smiled sarcastically at me. She probably though she was being criticised, but in fact she was the first person with nail varnish that I had ever seen.

This was not the only mistake that a nurse could make, even after several months training. Sister and staff nurse not being there, I was forced to answer the telephone on the ward one day and, since I was unsure of myself, I simply picked it up and said "hello" very gingerly into the mouthpiece. The sound of matron's quiet but decisive voice unnerved me even further.

"Don't hello to me," she told me down the phone, "Pick up the receiver, speak clearly and say 'this is ward whatever it is, Nurse whoever you are speaking, can I help you'- right? Now try it again."

So I did, and got it right, and never forgot it again.

The children's ward had its own ways quite separate from the adult wards. Of course, there was a lot more affection shown and physical contact made with the children; they had their own nightwear of pink or blue Vyella, lovely cuddly material for the poor little patients to wear. There was, however, an unpleasant task which was much more common in the children's ward as well – getting rid of head lice.

Children have always been very prone to infection from headlice, playing together as they do with close contact between their heads as they share a toy or book. To make sure that the child stayed free of lice after the adult headlice had been removed, Sassafras lotion was applied to the hair, then a cap was put on to cover the hair completely and finally a bandage was wrapped around the head to make sure the child could not scratch.

The child would feel very sorry indeed, and very ashamed too wearing this headgear – although there were so many of them they were hardly ever the only child wearing it. Also, the urge to scratch would sometimes drive them to tears and trying to rub their heads through the bandage picked up some of the lotion which was transferred to eyes and stung them too. All in all, the children were so relieved when they were clear of the lice and able to have their hair washed properly, that it was a treat to see them. The girls with long hair, which the nurses called 'nitty villas' because they so often harboured lice, were particularly glad to be rid of them because sister kept the ribbons from bouquets of flowers and tied up their clean, washed hair with bows to celebrate their victory when they were clear.

It was while I was on the children's ward that they heard they were to receive the honour of a visit from the King. King George V himself was going to be in Liverpool; he was going to visit the hospital and come to the ward to see the children. The routine of cleaning on the wards was very strict, but on the day the King was to come, the maids went into a positive frenzy of polishing, swinging the big 'dummy' as the polisher was called, back and forth across the floor until it shone. The children's toys were cleared off the beds and put away, the children were all in new pyjamas or nightgowns, washed and tidied until they were presentable – and then there was a delay, the King was late, he was held up elsewhere. The little patients became restless, more and more difficult to keep in their places, neat and tidy as they should be to meet a King, until finally the retinue arrived.

King George was all smiles as he progressed down the ward, and very kind to the children. At one point, he came over to speak to a lovely looking little African boy with big brown eyes and a mass of dark, curly hair.

"Hello, Johnny, how are you?" he enquired but instead of being suitably impressed by royalty the boy just turned away his head and scowled.

Sister was concerned, she told the child, "Tommy, answer His Majesty!", but the boy kept his lips firmly pressed together and would not respond.

The King, most kind and understanding, said, "Oh, your name is Tommy? I am sorry I got it wrong, will you speak to me now?" and at this the boy finally turned his head.

Everyone waited while he glowered around at the crowd of people by his bed, and he looked up to stare the King directly in the face, opened his mouth and told the King to 'bugger off'.

There was a sharp intake of breath from everyone else gathered around the bed, but thankfully, the King himself took it all in very good part and once he began to laugh, the other members of his retinue, and the nurses as well, could gratefully smile along with him, relieved that he had seen the funny side of it.

Another little boy, transferred from one of the other hospitals, arrived on a Sunday without his hospital notes. For quite a while, doctors and nurses could not understand what was the problem with the child. The small patient just cried, saying that Peter was sore. It was only when they realised that Peter was not his name, but in fact his penis, that they could settle him down and begin some treatment for him. Children were taught so many different names for the area of their body considered by parents to be 'not quite nice', that it was difficult to work out who was referring to what at times (even on the adult wards these euphemisms remained).

It was in the autumn that I joined the children's ward and in November the hospital, along with everyone else in Britain, prepared for Armistice Day. It was a simple matter of explaining to the children that at 11 a.m. on the 11th they must all be very quiet for a little while and try to think about all the brave people who had died for them in the War. It was a very special day for many adults who had lost friends or relatives in the War, but of course to the children it was just an ordeal, trying to keep quiet and still for two minutes. The nurses helped them by standing by bedsides and anyone who began to fidget was reminded by a finger to the lips or a shake of the head.

This was all working very well until one child with special difficulties, she was mentally disabled, was in fact using a bedpan at the time, decided she had had enough of all this silence and got off the bedpan, took off the top and began to dabble her hands in the contents, all the while crooning to herself "a-gee, a-gah, a-gee, a-gah" and rocking herself in time to her chant.

The sister glanced at the nurses who glanced at each other, and then with one accord they broke ranks and went over to the bed to prevent any further mishaps from the mentally retarded child. There were some things which came above even the solemn silence of Armistice Day and this was certainly one of them.

It was about this time, too, that a girl of about nine years old, who had had an appendectomy three days previously, began to feel very sick after eating her lunch. I brought her a bowl and held her head gently over the bowl, supporting her abdomen where the stitches were still rather new. Vomiting put a lot of strain on the abdomen and I didn't want the wound to burst. After a time, the girl really was sick, vomiting into the bowl and then both the girl and I recoiled in horror! There in the bowl was a twelve inch long white worm! Sister was called and she contacted the child's parents at once.

It turned out that the family had a dog, a favourite with the little girl – but a source of worm infection. The child playing out in the garden with her pet often ate mint straight from the garden, and cuddled and stroked her friend, all without washing her hands or the mint. So she had ingested the worm eggs which had grown inside her intestine until it had encountered the appendix. It had caused the appendix to become inflamed and the child had been brought into hospital for an appendectomy. The anaesthetic for the operation had disturbed the worm which was rejected by the child's stomach, to which the worm had travelled.

The parents were naturally horrified to hear of all this and at first their reaction was to have the dog destroyed to prevent any such thing happening again, but in fact the little girl's pet did not have to be put down. It had to be treated by a vet to get rid of the worm, of course, but once the child had learnt the simple hygiene rule (which she would stick to for the rest of her life) that you must always wash green vegetables before eating them and you must always wash your hands before putting them near your mouth, there was little chance of such a thing happening again.

Once, the children's ward was so full that a toddler with bronchopneumonia (which affected the young and the old) was put into a small cot bed in the female ward. I had fed the baby, changed her nappy and made her comfortable in the hope that she would settle down to sleep. The illness had taken a lot out of the little body and after a while she fell into a doze. I was pleased too, because while the child slept she was not in any pain and could regain some strength to help combat the disease. I was just relaxing my vigilance on the cot bed when another nurse went over to it and lifted the baby into a more upright position. The child woke immediately and began to cry loudly in distress.

I knew that the correct nursing position for a patient with pneumonia is in a semi-sitting position so that the fluid does not fill the lungs, but the baby had been sleeping quietly in a position only a little lower in the bed than that recommended and I had decided that the sleep was more important than the exact position as laid down in the book. Naturally, I was not pleased with this interference. So, after I had calmed the baby and settled her down again I took the other nurse along to the ward bathroom and there we exchanged a few words on the subject, after which I returned to the ward and my little patient.

On a lighter note, it was my first hospital Christmas in the children's ward. For weeks beforehand, the nurses and patients (those who could) were busy making paper garlands to decorate the ward. On the children's ward parents often brought in extras, presents and decorations, little treats to help ease the upset of Christmas in hospital. Also, many of the bigger firms in Liverpool sent in gifts suitable for the children's stockings.

It was just as well they did help out because each ward sister was given exactly £2 to provide for Christmas, including a tea for her staff on the ward on Christmas Day. The maids were off duty over Christmas but seven or eight nurses and one or two housemen would sit down in sister's room for tea. It was a help if a grateful patient had donated some money to the ward as well – presents for patients and decorations for the ward took up most of the £2 from the Hospital Committee, as each patient hung a stocking at the end of their bed.

The children (or those who were well enough to care about what time of year it was) had been very difficult to settle down the night before and on duty at 5.30 a.m. I was not surprised to find them waking up and clambering down the bed to check their stockings. Hung over the end of the beds the previous evening these stockings had now mysteriously been filled with little gifts and fruit. Once one child had found that Santa had visited them while they slept, all the ward was aroused by the cries and laughter, until pandemonium broke out up and down the beds, with the lights turned on and children opening their gifts.

Christmas Day was very special. A surgeon dressed in a white theatre gown would come round to carve the huge turkey which was wheeled into the ward on a trolley for all the patients to see. These turkeys weighed up to thirty pounds and while the surgeon carved one such monster in one ward, his registrar would be doing the same service in another. The trolleys were dressed very festively and then after the dinners were served the turkey was delivered back to the kitchen to make soup.

The nurses could not partake of this Christmas cheer, though. They were on duty and must remain so. It would be some days later that they had their own Christmas Dinner. They were waited on by senior staff and doctors and sisters alike, acting as waiters to keep the Christmas spirit going.

Unfortunately, one young houseman may have had too much Christmas spirit that first year. He was acting the fool with a soda syphon and one or two nurses got a very cold, soggy dinner indeed when he came up behind them and squirted them down the neck (and all over their plates on the table) in his exuberance.

Still, in general terms, Christmas was a good time. Even back in the Nurses' Home the girls gathered round in one of the rooms to eat a private feast of cake and biscuits sent from home. We were using our tooth mugs for cups, soap dishes for plates, and we were getting so much into the mood that we forgot to keep our voices down as we should have done. No food was allowed in the Nurses' Home and this was a strict rule. We were suddenly surprised by home sister coming up the corridor and opening the door which we had closed to conceal our feast.

We all froze, waiting to be told off in no uncertain terms indeed, but instead sister smiled around at us all, as we sat on the bed, or on the floor leant up against the washstand.

"Merry Christmas, nurses," she said, then added in a quiet voice, "Do try to keep the noise down, others are trying to sleep, remember."

Night Duty

Christmas feasts might take place in the Nurses' Home, but midnight feasts were unknown. The fact was that the nurses were too tired to stay awake if they had been on day duty whereas if they were on night duty they were too occupied on the ward.

The first time that I was given night duty I was told by my ward sister to go to second sitting at 1 p.m. for my dinner that day, then change my room. I already knew what this meant from talking to the other nurses so, after I had eaten, I went to my room in the Nurses' Home to gather up my personal things and my uniform. I packed them all into my suitcase and carried it back through the hospital. Outside, I turned up Hill Street, past the Anglican Cathedral which was in the process of being built, and walked on until I came to the hostel.

The hostel was in fact several old Georgian houses made into one large place to house those nurses from the Royal Southern Hospital who were on night duty at the time. Here the normal routine of things was entirely geared to night-time work, with meals and periods for rest all turned around to suit the nocturnal life. It made a lot of sense to separate them from the rest of the nurses; no-one had to beware of disturbing others trying to sleep in the middle of the day and everyone came and went together.

I arrived with my suitcase in my hand at the door of the hostel that first afternoon and knocked politely on the door. The sister in charge of the hostel must have been waiting for the new arrivals just inside the hallway because she opened the door almost at once and then stepped back to let me enter. Stepping quickly through into the dim hall from the comparative brightness of the daylight, I completely failed to see that there was a step as I entered the hostel and I tripped and measured my length on the polished hall.

Looking down calmly as both I and the suitcase skidded to a halt at her feet, sister remarked dryly, "Next time you come, nurse, walk in, don't slide." Embarrassed, I picked myself up, retrieved my suitcase and followed the sister to my new room. It was quite different from the room at the home, with large, light rooms divided up into cubicles for each nurse. Once I had unpacked and put away my things, I undressed and lay down on the bed to get a little rest. At 7 p.m. I knew I would be called by the maid to get up, get washed and dressed again and make my way with the others back down to the hospital for 'breakfast'. No meals were provided at the hostel, not even a cup of tea.

Another difference, which I noticed as I lay on the bed gazing across the room and out of the window, was the view. From my basement room in the Nurses' Home I had been able to see very little of the world, just rain or sunshine against the wall outside, but from this window I could see, even as I was lying back with my head on the pillow, the great stones being hauled up to build the new cathedral opposite.

The red sandstone blocks were being raised by hand using blocks and pulleys so there was very little noise to disturb me, just the voices of the men and the creaking of the ropes as the stones went up, followed by the chipping of chisels as they cut the stone once it had been manoeuvred into place. It was really quite soothing to watch, soporific in fact, and I felt myself drifting off to sleep – until, before I knew it, the maid was tapping at the door and I had to rouse myself to get back down to the hospital and be on duty at 8 p.m.

The sister at the hostel, the lady who had gazed down at me this afternoon, was quite an imposing figure even when seen from a standing position. She was very tall and had a deep voice. When she spoke to the nurses, she could be quite scathing at times and while she was never unkind, some of the nurses were a little wary of her dry wit.

After such an inauspicious entrance, I felt I could only improve the impression I might be making with sister, but in fact things went from bad to worse.

Shortly after I had begun my first three month spell of night duty, I was taking a bath when I found out something fundamental about the bathroom at the hostel. It contained a large cylinder full of boiling water to provide plenty of hot baths for the girls. This made a wonderful place to drape towels and night dresses so that they were warm. I had pulled a hot towel off the cylinder and was busily drying my feet when a slight wobble due to standing on one foot to dry the other caused me to back into the exposed cylinder. I cried out and jumped away as soon as I realised what had happened but the damage was done. The bare flesh on my bottom had stuck to the hot metal, and when I bounded away from the cylinder I left two patches of skin behind.

Without a further thought, I rushed out of the bathroom and dashed through the sitting-room past the amazed faces of my friends to get to sister's room for help. Imagine my chagrin to find sister in the process of entertaining two visitors (ladies, thankfully). I stopped short at the door and blurted out my tale of woe. The visitors might stare at the sight of me dressed only in a towel standing in the doorway in obvious distress but sister simply raised an eyebrow and seemed not at all interested.

"Well, I suppose you won't do that again, will you," was all she said in reply to the explanation of what had happened, and she was right. I never did do it again. At the time, however, I only felt very sorry for myself as I made my way back to the bathroom to retrieve my clothes and dress my own wounds.

For days afterwards, it was very sore indeed to sit down or stand up. Each movement opened up the raw area of the burns again and the healing was slow because of this. I had to go about my duties just as usual, wincing each time I moved, instead of resting the wounds to give them time to recover. They did eventually heal, though.

When I set off with the other night duty nurses to go down the hill to the hospital, it often struck me what a strange little group we made. We always wore our capes and our caps and each of us carried a bag or a bundle of books for our studies, and often some knitting or sewing to be done in the quiet hours of the night. It wasn't long before I joined the ranks of those nurses who also packed their carpet slippers. When night sister had finished her rounds of the wards at about 10 p.m. the nurses knew they would be able to slip on their slippers to ease their aching feet for a few hours before they had to put their shoes back on in readiness for her next visit.

When we reached the hospital we picked up our billy-cans with our 'dinner' in. Each night duty nurse was expected to make her own meal in the ward kitchen at midnight because the cooks went home at the end of the day. We soon learned not to hope for much from these billy-cans. There would be a sausage and a potato, both raw, or perhaps an egg instead of the sausage, also raw. From such unpromising ingredients, we had to make an edible meal. This challenge showed the nurses' sense of initiative as we did our best to make something from the extremely basic things provided.

Olive oil, which was kept on the ward for medicinal purposes such as rubbing into the skin to help prevent bedsores, could be used to fry an egg or a sausage, or even a few chips. Bengers food, a powdered product used to make a nutritious liquid diet, and would make a reasonable pancake mix when combined with an egg.

Using my raw egg and a little milk I made myself an egg custard one night in the ward kitchen on the children's ward. I heated the custard using the double saucepan principle, with a stone jar and a pan which was kept in the kitchen for heating up water to warm the babies' bottles – but I never found out how my improvised meal tasted, although it smelt very good indeed.

I had to leave it in the kitchen for quite a while because I was nursing three babies with meningitis, all of whom were very ill. Each spasm of pain brought on a distinctive cry from the child and arching of the body. I was completely taken up with my patients for quite a while until they gradually settled down to sleep for some of the night. Once they were asleep, I was free to go and get my custard from the kitchen. It was about 1 a.m. and I was feeling really ready for my meal but when I went to check the jar I found that the other, less welcome, residents of the hospital had got to it first. The rats had been busy and licked the jar clean.

As I sterilised the jar before putting it away, I reflected that I should have known by now that I ought to have put a cover of some sort, preferably a heavy one, on the jar when I left the kitchen. Although they were seldom seen, everyone knew the rats were there. It was only to be expected with the hospital situated as it was in the dock area of a large seaport. The place was kept spotlessly clean but still the vermin would come in after any scraps of food left around. This was in part why the nurses were not permitted any food in the home or the hostel. It would have invited rats in there as well. The hospital also suffered from cockroaches and steam flies which crept in wherever they could find a crack.

On the night I lost my custard to the rats, I did not in fact see any of the creatures. They were remarkable for their bold behaviour yet were very seldom seen. If no-one had been in the kitchen for a while, and then somebody went in quickly and turned on the light, you would see them running along the plate-racks of the dresser and whisking along by the skirting-boards for a moment or two until suddenly they were gone. In the middle of a long night duty their scurrying noises were often quite loud to a nurse with ears tuned to the quiet of the ward.

On another night duty on a different ward I had no time to listen out for rats. Nursing a patient with lobar pneumonia – which affected young adults, rather than the bronchopneumonia which mainly hit the elderly and the very young – I was kept busy again during the early part of the night as the young man's temperature climbed and the crisis approached. Ice compresses to the forehead, cold drinks, tepid sponging of the body, all in an effort to keep his temperature down, occupied my time until the restless tossing and laboured breathing reached a peak. Then the temperature dropped suddenly, the breathing became easier, the patient less distressed. The crisis was over, the patient would begin to recover from this time onward.

As my patient slipped into a quiet sleep, I tidied away the bowl of water, the compresses and cloths, and returned to sit by the bedside in case I was needed further. All was peaceful, I was tired and the young man slept soundly. Suddenly, into this silence came the jingle-jangle of a rising series of notes on the piano that stood at the far end of the ward. I was shaken out of my reverie, in fact I nearly had a crisis myself. Turning quickly, I saw a large rat plop down off the end of the piano keyboard and hurry away into the gloom. "Not waiting for the applause," I thought as I went to close the cover over the keys. None of the patients had been disturbed, only I myself had heard the moonlight sonata and in future, although I knew the day staff were supposed to shut it, I glanced across the room to make sure that the piano lid was firmly down when I came on duty at night.

The strangest sight I ever saw on night duty was one dark evening on the orthopaedic ward. Sitting at the table with the lamp creating a pool of light just around me and nowhere else, I looked up to see an apparition approaching down the length of the ward. A ghostly shape in white was all that I could make out for a moment, until the swarthy-skinned man grinned at me and I saw the light reflecting from his smile and in his eyes. He had an arm abducted out at right angles to his body and this and the white nightshirt had formed a weird unnatural shape not immediately recognisable as a person at all.

During the long nights alone on the ward at about 2 a.m. everyone was at their lowest ebb. The nurses might have brought study books or knitting to pass the time at the ward table with the desk lamp on but by 2 a.m. learning or needlework had lost their charms and it was quite a fight to keep alert. Night sister had done her round earlier and administered any medicines needed, but she often came round again probably because she knew the nurses left alone, one to each ward, would be feeling at their sleepiest and she wanted to make sure they did not doze.

I did not mind sister visiting the ward and asking how everyone was, but sometimes sister checked up on individual patients as well, any of them who were very ill, or seemed particularly restless. This she did by shining a torch into their faces and asking them if they were asleep! Now, I knew that those who were properly asleep would not be woken by this treatment, but the patients who were lightly dozing would be jerked awake by the light and it was up to the nurse in charge of the ward to settle them down again once sister had left.

Luckily, I had a very good method of settling them down. I would make a cup of tea for them and one for myself as well and then the two of us, patient and I, would have a little chat while tea was being drunk. This helped the patient to get off to sleep again and I was refreshed and ready to carry on my duties. The cups had to be removed and washed before sister came round again though, because such little things were not strictly allowed. We were not allowed to sit by the bedside even to feed the patient.

The responsibility of being in charge of thirty beds for the night was heavy. Apart from sister's rounds, there was one extra nurse between every four wards and she was sent round to spend half an hour in each ward to help with lifting or other tasks. Otherwise, the nurse was on her own with the patients.

On one occasion I was asked to keep an eye on a man who had been brought in through casualty as a morphine addict. I was told to keep him under observation for the night and I and another nurse had to stand by as he was undressed and put into a hospital nightshirt to make sure he was 'clear' of all drugs and syringes. We both watched him very carefully as we helped him to strip and get into bed. After a while he appeared to go to sleep.

Later I returned from the ward kitchen I realised he had not been asleep at all. I found him trying to open the drugs cupboard. It was as well that the nurses carried the keys in their pockets because if the key had been on the table the man would undoubtedly have opened the cupboard and taken the morphine that was in there. He had a syringe in his hand ready to use and I could only marvel at how he must have transferred it from his clothes to the bed while being watched the whole time by myself and the other nurse. Needless to say, he was transferred the next day to a more secure place.

It was assumed that the night duty would be quiet and therefore the nurse had also to prepare the breakfast for the patients ready to waken them in the morning. The trolleys had to be set up with everything ready and there was a 4lb loaf to cut each morning in the ward kitchen. Now, for some reason, every knife in the hospital was blunt and the bread knives were the bluntest. I hated the mess and hard work involved in getting that loaf cut into even the thickest of doorstep slices. I had been brought up with sharp knives and neat, thin slices of bread, and so, with a little of my small amount of savings I went out and bought a brand new bread knife. I brought this into the hospital on my next night duty and early the following morning I could be heard merrily slicing my way with no trouble at all through the big, crusty loaf.

I could be heard, all right. I was heard by sister on her rounds who came to investigate the loud and unwarranted noise. Apparently, in the quiet of the sleeping hospital the sound of bread being sliced was echoing down the corridors and annoying people trying to sleep! sister confiscated that sharp, new knife and I had to be content once more with hacking the loaves laboriously into pieces half an inch thick or more.

The patients never seemed to mind their hunks of bread. They didn't mind their hard boiled eggs either. Each morning some would ask for their egg to be 'lightly boiled, please, nurse'. Each morning the eggs were put into the big pan of boiling water, thirty of them, one after another, and which one went in first was always impossible to tell. So each morning the patients got their eggs hard or soft boiled by luck and by lottery – but they never really complained.

At the end of the night, each nurse handed over to the ward sister. This meant reporting on all her patients, how they had been during the night. It had to be done in the proper manner, standing in front of sister with cuffs on and cap and uniform neat, no matter how tired I was at that time. Then, after handing back my billy-can and having breakfast in the refectory, I left the hospital to walk back up the hill to the hostel with the other night nurses, come hail, rain or snow.

It gave me sympathy with all night workers as I returned each morning, sometimes in summer when the early day was a delight to be out in, sometimes in winter when it was cold and dark and wet. It was a strange feeling of topsy-turvy, with my suitcase of study books (and bedroom slippers), as I hurried back to bed, having watched the dawn come up from the window of the children's ward, or switched off the lights in casualty and said good morning to the day staff coming on duty.

Casualty and Clinics

Night duty sometimes took me into the casualty department. This was where the nurses met the public head-on, not as a patient already admitted to a ward but just as they came in off the street.

One of the things they did not have time to do with some of the admissions was to wash them. They might be ill but they certainly were not clean and very often they might, like the children on the children's ward, have unwelcome visitors, lice or fleas, that were particularly discouraged in a hospital where hygiene was so very important.

At first, I found myself playing host to a flea or two (which was quickly despatched) but after a while I found that a good rub of camphorate oil around the collar and cuff deterred them. Then it was back to the problem of removing them from the patients if they were to be admitted to the wards.

One old lady who was being cleaned and ready to be admitted to hospital was quite happy to be stripped, to have her clothes taken away for cleansing and to have her hair and body washed in a warm bath. Quite happy, that is, until I tried to wash out her umbilicus. Then she squirmed, she objected, she refused. Her belly-button, the place where God pressed in the dough to see if each new-made human was done, was not to be touched. She had never washed in that little knot in her entire life (and she was quite old) because, if she did, then the knot might come undone!

It took a lot of persuasion to convince the woman that she would come to no harm if she cleaned out her navel, but eventually I did it.

The evening shift in casualty could turn up some strange occurrences indeed. Sometimes the night would be very busy with admissions from a street fight after the pubs closed, a road accident when pedestrians were difficult to see in the dark, or on one occasion a tram accident when a tram had jumped the rails and the passengers were injured.

On such a night the doctor might well not have any time to spare for the young lads who delighted in coming into casualty to pester them with mock injuries, but when things were slack he would deal with them as well.

I, who had never met this sort of behaviour before, was mystified to find the doctor taking seriously a claim from a boy of about seventeen that he had swallowed a mouse. I listened in puzzlement as the doctor advised the lad to come into a cubicle and lie down and I frowned in surprise when I was told to go to housekeeping sister to get a small piece of cheese. Nevertheless, as I had been instructed by a doctor, I did as I was told and returned after some discussion with housekeeping sister with a very small piece of hard cheddar cheese in my hand. It was like asking for gold, who? why? was it needed?

"Right, Nurse, put the cheese down there on the pillow next to his head," the doctor told me and then solemnly addressed the boy who was lying flat on his back looking up at them from the bed. "Now, lad, you turn your head to the side facing the cheese, open your mouth and then – keep very, very still and in an hour or two the smell of the cheese should entice that mouse right back up."

Taking me by the arm, the doctor walked smartly out of the cubicle and left the practical joker to himself. In about five minutes time the lad emerged from the cubicle and slunk sheepishly away. "There's one that won't be back," the doctor said, and some weeks later he demonstrated again how to discourage pranksters.

This time a youngster had decided to embarrass the nurses by coming in clutching his abdomen and crying out that he couldn't pass his water. He supposed that this would cause alarm but the doctor must have seen him before and knew him for a scamp. Again, he led the boy to a cubicle and asked him to lie on the bed. Then, with a wink at me, he turned away to a cupboard and took out a cystoscope. This large, metal instrument, which he showed in great detail to the lad, would now be passed up from the outside into his bladder in order to view the bladder internally and see what was the trouble. He then requested the boy to undo his trousers so we could proceed.

As expected, the patient leapt down from the bed and ran out of the hospital, never to bother them again.

How the doctor could tell the fakers from the genuine people, I just did not know, but I found that others too could have their suspicions of something not quite right with a situation.

A man had been picked up as a drunk by the police. He had been falling down in the street, his speech slurred and he was slipping into what appeared to be a drunken stupor but when they took him back to the cells at the police station, the police were not happy that he was just simply drunk. They decided to bring him to casualty which proved to be a very good decision indeed. The man was not drunk at all. He was a diabetic who was passing gradually into a diabetic coma and their prompt action saved his life. American doctors Banting and Best had discovered insulin in 1929 and from that time onward, diabetes could be treated.

I took part in some of the early work on the electrocardiograph. Dr Noble Chamberlain, a heart specialist working in Liverpool, was trying to record the activity of the heart on paper. The nurses in the hospital were happy to volunteer as guinea pigs and sit with their hands and feet in saline baths while wired up to his machine. The work he did enabled doctors from that time on to make a permanent record of the rhythm of the heart instead of only listening to it. Much progress has of course been made in the medical field since those days.

Two other patients brought into casualty after the case of the diabetic man were two small children, five or six years old, who proved to be really drunk. They were staggering about, quite disorientated, and very unhappy with the way they felt. They were even more unhappy when they had to have their stomachs washed out and they let everyone know about it.

They went to sleep after a while, though, watched over by me, and the parents and relatives who had brought them in explained in more detail how it had happened. It seemed that they were all taking refreshments back at the house after attending a family funeral when someone noticed that the children had been helping themselves to the dregs from everyone's glasses. Of course for such small children this had been more than enough to cause acute alcohol poisoning.

In the morning the children were allowed home. They did not in fact have much of a hangover because most of the alcohol had been removed from their stomachs, but they were very subdued little teetotallers just the same.

A far worse self-inflicted poisoning case came in one night for me to deal with. A young girl, a redhead, had become an opium addict. This was not as unusual as it might seem. There was a street, Pitt Street, near the docks in Liverpool, which was known to be an opium den area. The Chinese sailors frequented it, along with many others, unfortunately, and the street was one which I had been told to avoid. Whatever the original reason, this girl had been ensnared by the drug and had been prostituting herself in the opium dens to get more. She had been thrown out into the street when she became too ill to be of any use to the men there any more.

I could not imagine what could bring a girl not much older than myself to such a state, but I did know that I must keep the girl awake all through the night as to fall asleep in her condition could prove fatal to her. It was a hard task. Everything inside her was telling the girl to lie down and sleep, to let go and float away – perhaps never to return. Conversation about the weather, the time of the year, family, nursing, even football, failed to make any impression on the girl. She remained surly, unhelpful and ungrateful – but awake. I passed her over to the day staff with a sigh of relief.

It was in the casualty department too that I saw my first baby delivered. A woman had been brought in on the point of delivery. In the hustle and bustle of the birth, I was handed the baby, a very small, premature child, and told to wrap it up quickly to keep it warm. I looked around for the nearest thing to wrap this little scrap in and, seeing a roll of cottonwool, I used that. It seemed ideal; soft, warm and hygienic. The only problem, which I discovered to my cost a little later on, was that the fluffy wisps of the cottonwool had stuck to the baby and would not come off.

When a baby is in the womb it is covered by a protective sticky substance called the vernix. This prevents the unborn skin from becoming waterlogged. Inside the amniotic sac the baby floats in a watery fluid and the vernix stops this fluid reaching the skin. Once the baby is born, the first wash removes this sticky layer, but in the meantime I had wrapped this particular baby in the cottonwool which had stuck fast. The baby looked like a new-born lamb in its soft white coat! Fortunately, the cottonwool was eventually removed along with the vernix when the baby was washed. There were no incubators in those days, just tender loving care.

The other places where nurses met the public just as they walked in from the street were the outpatients clinics and it was here that I moved next.

Casualty had been a very mixed bag; never knowing what would be the problem with the next patient to arrive – anything from birth to death could take place in one day or night. Outpatients was quite a different matter altogether. Each batch of patients was there to see a particular consultant and therefore they all had the same area of complaint. Perhaps their eyes, perhaps their joints, perhaps a skin problem. Whatever it was, they were grouped accordingly and seen by the ophthalmic surgeon, the ear nose and throat surgeon, the dermatologist, etcetera, each one to his own speciality.

A nurse could be moved from one clinic to another as she was needed but I soon got to know some of the regular visitors to outpatients. One person who never attended a clinic but was talked about quite often as the patients swapped ailments in the waiting area was a gentleman called Arthur Rightus! Nearly everyone at the orthopaedic clinic seemed to know him – "it's me Arthur Rightus, you know," they would tell each other in confidence. If Arthur could have been sent packing, thought I, there would have been a lot less people attending the clinic!

At the orthopaedic clinic I made the acquaintance of a very grumpy sour woman, who perhaps had something to be grumpy about as she had brittle bones, but who nevertheless was a positive pain to the nurses as they tried to cheer her up. She had come down for physiotherapy because she had broken her femur. She was recovering on the female surgical ward but needed exercises and massage to keep the muscles of her leg strong. It was simply bad luck that she fell while walking down to the department and it was only to be expected that, suffering from osteoporosis as she did, she broke her other thigh when she fell. She had almost recovered from her original fracture but now the second leg had to be put into a Thomas splint instead and she was put back in the ward to recover once again. The nurses were less than pleased to see her back again for another long stay. She was quite simply impossible to please. If she were give a cup of tea, it was too hot or too cold, too sweet or not sweet enough, and when she continued to complain even when given the sugar bowl and invited to serve herself, the nurses had their patience sorely tried to keep a pleasant face for her.

Like her or lump her, they nursed her for another few weeks until it was time to take off the splint. The Thomas splint was used to immobilise a leg and keep it straight and steady so that the bones could knit properly. Before plaster of Paris was used, this apparatus of metal tubes and webbing straps was used on all leg fractures. The patient had to stay in bed whilst the splint was on the leg. Once the splint was removed, the woman was supposed to stay in bed unless assisted to get out but, perhaps her pillows weren't straight, or maybe she wanted to complain about the tea again. Whatever the reason, she tried to get out of bed herself and fell. Naturally enough, for a woman with her condition a fall from a high sided hospital bed was certain to cause another broken bone and it did. She broke her other leg! That is to say, she broke the leg which had been broken first, before she broke the other one.

When the consultant orthopaedic surgeon saw her, he gazed at her in disbelief. "Woman," he said, "it's a good thing you're not a ruddy centipede!" and he shook his head in sorrow.

Another orthopaedic surgeon, Sir Robert Jones, who was getting on in years but sometimes came to the hospital to visit his colleagues, was responsible for inventing an abduction frame which was named after him. This frame was another method of stretching and immobilising the limbs while they healed. There was always a flurry of excitement and reverence when the great man came round.

A woman arrived for a clinic one morning with the usual sample of urine in a bottle. These were often requested by the doctor and would be brought along, collected and labelled by the nurse, and sent off to the laboratory for tests. On this occasion, as I was marking up a label with the name of the patient, the woman remarked conversationally, "It ain't mine this morning, nurse. I only remembered I was supposed to bring it after I'd been – so I've brought you me hubby's instead."

Working on the eye clinic, the nurse had quite a routine to follow. The consultant required the pupils of the eyes to be as wide open as possible so that he could see well inside the eye and for this purpose the nurse had to administer atropine drops onto the eyes of each patient before they were examined. These drops caused the pupils to dilate and then after the examination some esserine drops were put onto the eye to counteract the effects of the atropine.

Having explained this routine to one lady, I put on the first drops and the consultant began his examination. After this was completed, I shepherded the woman through into the recovery room and asked her to wait there for the second, counteracting, drops. After I had taken the next patient into the consultant and having put atropine drops onto his eyes, I returned to the recovery room to find the woman had gone! I was very concerned and quickly went to the door to see if I could call the woman back but there was not sign of her. I was most worried about the effect of the atropine on this woman – I knew that without the esserine drops to return her to normal, she would be suffering temporarily from tunnel vision and not realise that her sight was impaired.

I sent one of the porters, who were always in attendance at the clinics, out into the street to search for the woman but without success. It bothered me for the rest of the clinic, I felt I ought to have been able to do something to stop the woman leaving, although I knew really that I could not have done. I could not be in two places at once.

In this case, my fears were in fact realised. Not more than an hour later an ambulance arrived at casualty with the very same woman inside. She had walked to the nearest tram stop, caught a tram to the centre of Liverpool, planning to go shopping at Lewis's Department Store, but when she stepped down from the tram she had completely misjudged the distance because of the effect of the drops on her eyes. The trams stopped in the middle of the road, on their tram tracks and in stepping awkwardly into the road the woman had failed to see a car coming and had fallen badly, been hit by a glancing blow, and broken her leg.

It stayed with me for some time thinking that it had been 'my fault' that this had happened and despite being aware that it was in fact a freak accident, I spent the rest of my time on the eye clinic making sure that no-one ever 'got away' again.

Whenever an X-ray was needed, the sister in outpatients or on the ward would take the patient down to the basement of the hospital where the X-ray equipment was kept. There were no lead-lined aprons at this time. No-one had any idea there was any danger from X-rays and quite happily stayed by the patient each time an X-ray was taken.

Throughout my period in outpatients, I was impressed by the sister there. The sisters in every department were very good, of course, as only the best were asked to stay on and continue their careers with the hospital but this particular sister was very strict while remaining very kind as well.

It was Christmas time again by the time I had come round to outpatients, so with the clinics stopped over Christmas for a few days the sister closed the department. After tidying the cupboards and leaving everything spick and span for the New Year, the nurses were sent around the wards to help out and entertain the patients. Some of the nurses sang, some of them did the can-can, they helped put up decorations and generally joined in the fun. Then on Christmas Eve they went from ward to ward with lanterns, singing carols with the other nurses and the patients.

It was after this that the nurses from outpatients went back with sister to her room to have tea with her, a very great privilege for them, and afterwards they asked her to tell them about her experiences nursing during the Great War in the Queen Alexandra Royal Army Nursing Corps. She was fascinating to listen to, a really interesting person. The nurses went back to the Nurses' Home that evening full of renewed dedication to nursing and admiration for such a lady.

It was a tragedy that this sister, before the next Christmas came round, had died of a simple illness – but so often this was the case, the simplest cold could develop into pneumonia, a wound could become infected, or a fever rage through a body and someone you knew well could die. It was sometimes, perhaps, because of this very uncertainty of life that people became nurses, to try to help in the fight against pain and death.

Exams

All through our three years' training, the probationer nurses were expected to study hard and absorb knowledge both on the wards and in the lecture rooms. These lecture rooms were in the Nurses' Home.

A lecture took place when it suited the lecturer, be they consultant, hygiene officer, or sister tutor. The last people whose convenience was considered when scheduling a lecture were the probationer nurses. If a lecture was at 3 p.m. in the afternoon, then any nurses who were on night duty had to get up in the middle of their 'night,' get dressed and walk down from the hostel to the hospital. There they took their places in the lecture-room, trying to keep awake and pay attention to the teacher. No-one dreamed of changing the times of lectures to suit these unfortunate girls, yawning and blinking as they tried to learn.

Naturally, after struggling to stay alert for an hour or more, they had neither the time nor the inclination to go back up the hill to the hostel and undress again in order to have an hour or so's sleep. They found their way instead to the sitting-rooms in the Nurses' Home and there they would study their books, write up notes from the lecture they had just attended, or perhaps try to snatch a few minutes dozing in one of the easy chairs by the fire. (As well as any probationers on night duty, any nurse unlucky enough to have an afternoon or a day off when she had to attend a lecture had to cancel any plans for that day and stay at the hospital for the lecture).

There was always something to learn on the wards as well. Nurses were taught a great deal just by assisting a qualified nurse or staff nurse or the sister on a ward. Gradually as the months went by, they were asked to do more and more by themselves, gaining their experience by practical means backed up by the theory of the classroom in those occasional lectures. In fact, it was on the wards that most of the teaching took place. They had to write notes, and study their textbooks at all times while still working a twelve hour day. On night duty, the nurses would carry their books with them and spend many an hour leaning close to the pages in the light of the desk lamp while all the rest of the ward was in semi-darkness.

They were expected to pass an examination at the end of eighteen months, and another at the end of their three years' training. If any nurse failed either of these exams she was able to try again once more, but no more than that. If she didn't come through, or indeed if she decided at any time that she had made a mistake and nursing was not for her, then she must look elsewhere for her career. In the time that I was training, there were one or two girls who just did not fit into the dedicated, disciplined life and these very soon packed their bags and left.

Far more sad were the girls who wanted to succeed but couldn't manage the exams. Nerves, or lack of study, or some other reason could sometimes thin the ranks. 'There, but for the grace of God, go I,' thought the other nurses and spent yet more of their spare time reading and comparing notes in the sitting-room each evening. This was a rare occurrence, though, and none of my colleagues failed.

When I first started my training, there seemed to me to be an exam looming on the horizon all the time, because the older girls were constantly cramming themselves with extra knowledge for some imminent test or other. After a while, however, I began to see that because of the way the year was arranged at the hospital, there were three separate lots of exams each year. In the months of February, June and October there was a new intake of students and therefore the Preliminary exams at eighteen months and the Finals at three years came round at these times as well.

I took my Prelims, as they were known, in October 1929. I had studied hard and worked in the various different wards. My parents had paid the £2 entrance fee for me. Now, whatever the exams were like, I hoped I would do well for their sake as well as my own. In actual fact, the tests were a mixture of written work and practical, just like the training itself. There were three papers to answer, anatomy, physiology and hygiene. A surgeon marked the first, a physician the second and the matron or a tutor sister marked the third. These papers took about two hours and then there was the practical in the afternoon. Firstly, the nurses (all with numbers rather than names to identify them so that there would be no prejudice) had twenty minutes oral examination by a surgeon, a physician, a tutor sister, and two matrons (not their own) or sister tutors. Each examiner had a separate room to interview the nurse and then they came out into the larger practical room.

This was set out like part of a ward and there were two patients awaiting some sort of treatment. The convalescent patients loved to take part in these tests and if they knew the nurses they would smile encouragingly at them when they came in. Also in the room were tables set up with the equipment for various procedures. The nurse was then asked to carry out first one treatment and then another, all under the critical gaze of the matron or sister tutor examiner.

After an hour of this, the nurse was free to go. Free to carry on with her duties, that is, until some weeks later when she heard the results of the exams. I remembered little of the exams themselves but I remembered very well the feeling of pleasure when I heard that I had passed. There were only two results for each section of an examination – pass or fail. The nurses were not given a mark or a grade for any subject, just told if they had failed that they would have to sit that subject again. My family were the first to know, of course, and they were so proud of my achievements to date that I became quite embarrassed on my trips home when visitors were shown all the photographs of me in uniform and told of my progress, month by month.

After the strain of exams, it was a relief to take an occasional day off and go with friends into the city centre. After a good look round the shops; Reeces was always favourite; we would treat ourselves to a Devonshire cream tea in the Lyceum tea rooms at 1/6d each. Adding to this extravagance, we would sometimes queue for an hour or more to get a 1/3d ticket for the 'Gods' at the Empire Theatre. Once inside, we climbed the stairs until we were dizzy with the height – our seats were so far up that we felt that we might fall right down on to the stage if we leaned too far forward over the rail in front. We then watched a variety show, or play, or a musical, it didn't really matter what it was, it was the treat of being there that was such fun. It cost 1/3d in old money.

When we went back to the Nurses' Home after such a frivolous day, we felt refreshed to begin again the hard work and dedication to the patients that we needed in the hospital. It was a real safety valve for us all.

On our way to and from the centre of town, we had to walk through a great many poor streets but strangely we never felt threatened or ill at ease. The housewives in these streets kept themselves and their houses as clean as new pins, the steps were scrubbed and whitened and the ladies themselves would stand passing the time of day with their neighbours after washing down the pavement in front of their house, each woman in a clean white apron and a shawl. The children too were fond of the nurses and the wickedest of little urchins would offer to carry the bag of any nurse passing by in her uniform, such was the esteem in which they were held. Neither did the men molest them, although some of the dock workers and sailors around Hill Street were the poorest of the poor. Still, whether they were leaning in doorways or sitting on steps, they never had a thing to say to make a nurse blush as she hurried past on her way to the hospital. These men lived a wretched life, without a home of their own. The hostels in Hill Street and the surrounding area were dirty and mean – one charged 3d for board and blanket. Not bed and board, but just what it said! The man was given a pillow, a blanket and a board to lie on for his 3d, and in the morning he was turned out again.

Many of the sailors were foreign, passing the time until the next ship that would take them. I saw so many foreigners both in the streets and in the hospital that I soon became familiar with African faces, Asian faces, Eastern European faces, faces from all around the world. The tattooed lady in the women's ward and the little boy who told King George to "bugger off" were just two more patients to the Royal Southern Hospital.

Compared to some of these, the nurses were well paid, but by most standards they were not. It always made me smile when pay day came around to see the elaborate ritual which surrounded such a small payment. Two men arrived at the hospital with the money and a large ledger. They sat behind a table accompanied by the assistant matron who was there to identify each nurse for them as the nurses came to the table. The ledger lay open in front of them and when a nurse was given her pay it was solemnly marked off in the book. All this for a sum of £15 in the first year, doled out in quarterly amounts of £3 (the balance of £3 going towards insurance, superannuation and any breakages during the year)!

In the second year, the probationers got a salary of £30, in the third year £45 and if they were lucky enough to be asked to stay on as a staff nurse then they would receive the princely sum of £75 and think themselves very well off indeed. Perhaps some of the poor souls sleeping in the hostels, or trying to feed a family in one of the little terraced houses near the hospital would have agreed with that sentiment, and with no sense of irony about it either. When I considered that my bed and board were provided, my food (although not good) was always adequate for me, my uniform was washed, and my room cleaned for me, I realised that I had a lot to be thankful for, despite always feeling tired from the work. I even managed to put a little money aside for savings – sixpence or a shilling every three months in the post office despite the occasional extravagant trip into town.

Of course, out of this money had to come any extras in the way of fares home, days out, shopping, etc. Also, around Christmas time we were expected to contribute to the cost of a present for staff nurse and sister and the other nurses, including night staff, on the ward. 7/6d for sister, 5/- for staff nurse, 2/6d for the other nurses. This made quite a hole in the £3 quarterly pay and little else for relatives!

Nevertheless, when I received a wedding invitation from a relative, I was determined to buy an outfit for myself because I had nothing at all suitable to wear. Naturally, however, I knew I must look for the cheapest possible way to get one. I knew of a convalescent patient in the women's surgical ward who was a seamstress and who was pleased to be asked to make up a suit for a nurse, provided she was given the material. I took a trip into town, visited Lewises and bought a length of red cloth, which I took back to the hospital and presented to the woman straight away. The seamstress's face told me I had made a mistake. This material was very soft, not really suitable for a costume, I was told. As there was nothing to be done about it, the cut length of material could hardly be taken back, I just told her to get on with it, I was sure it would be all right – but it wasn't!

The red colour itself called attention to the suit and this made me feel uncomfortable as soon as I put it on, but when my parents first set eyes on it at the wedding they simply stood and stared in horror. The suit creased. It creased very badly, and that was really all you could say about it. It was not a success. I wished I had been permitted to attend the wedding in my uniform. It would have looked so much smarter, but we were never permitted to wear uniform outside the hospital. One good thing to come from this episode was that my parents were kind enough to pay for a new wool suit for me in a sensible navy fleck which lasted me for quite a few years. I supposed that the idea of their daughter wearing the crumpled red suit in public again was just too much for them. Whatever the reason, my mother wasted no time in getting me fitted out, she came to Liverpool to meet me on my very next day off to see it!

The half day off each week was never enough to plan a real outing. If we were lucky (and home sister had not stripped back the bed in their room in the Nurses' Home because she did not approve of the way it had been made up) we could slip into town by wearing brown stockings under the regulation black ones to save time in changing, rushing back to our rooms to change out of uniform – nurses were not allowed into town in uniform – and then hurrying to catch a bus. It hardly seemed worth the bother to me sometimes, the whole afternoon was a mad scramble, either to get into town or to get home to Fleetwood if I had the money for the fare.

Far more enjoyable were the full days off spent either with some of the other nurses or occasionally visiting relatives or friends of the family who lived in Liverpool. Two of my elderly aunts were shocked one afternoon when during tea at their houses, I calmly shook the tea off my teaspoon and used it to eat my boiled egg! How could they know that in the hospital, teaspoons were the first item of cutlery to go missing from a set and therefore every nurse kept her own personal spoon in her pocket at all times? They simply thought that their brother's child was very badly brought up indeed.

In fact, cutlery was so precious at the hospital that the nurses had to count it every day. Each ward's allocation was laid out on the table in the ward kitchen and checked every evening. Each week the assistant matron would come to see that noting had gone astray. Apart from the cost of any replacement knives or forks having to be met out of the voluntary funds, there was also the risk of cutlery finding its way into the pig bins with the waste food. The contents were paid for and taken away by a farmer for use as pigswill and if one of his pigs had died as a result of swallowing a teaspoon, the hospital would have found itself liable to pay for the animal. The nurses had to search the bins and the patient's lockers if any items of cutlery were lost, although sometimes they were not successful. One gentleman was thrilled to find himself back in Albert ward for a second time since he had only had time to collect five spoons on the previous visit and wanted to complete his set! Naturally, he was discouraged, and watched most carefully for any further signs of pilfering.

Some friends of my Gran's that I went to see on several afternoons over the three years of my training were very sweet and always tried to feed me well, knowing perhaps about the poor diet in the hospital. One meal I could never forget was not such a good one though. Somehow, some soap had got into the pan, perhaps falling in when the pan was filled with water, or being put in with the potatoes after it had fallen into the sink amongst the peelings. However it had got there, it made the potatoes taste truly awful. The old couple didn't seem to notice anything, however, so perhaps I had been served with the only piece. I decided to keep quiet for fear of hurting their feelings but it was a real effort to eat my meal and I refused all offers of a second helping.

The old gentleman always insisted on escorting me back to the hospital after my visits to them, despite my protestations that no-one ever annoyed the nurses as they came and went about their business. He would take me right to the front steps of the hospital and leave me there with a lift of his hat as he started back home himself.

The best days were the days I went home, though. My parents and my sisters were always glad to see me, the food was exactly what I liked and my place was there for me, as comfortable back in the family as if I had never left it. How strange it was to return from one way of life to the other, now that I had grown used to the nursing life!

During my final year, I took part in a collection for the hospital. sixty nurses were taken to Liverpool Cotton Exchange and formed up into a living S.O.S. on the flagstones there. Then each pair of nurses was given two envelopes and sent off to various businesses to collect money. Every office seemed to know we were coming and at the first stop my companion and I were handed a cheque straight away. Our second collection was from Reeces cafe where we were given a good dinner and then handed another cheque to take back with us as we made our own way back to the hospital.

This was one of the ways that money was raised on a regular basis. There was an organisation called Friends of the Royal Southern which also arranged collections and whose members gave money of their own towards the upkeep of the hospital. The whole thing was run on charity and budgeted very tightly because of that. They could not waste the funds so generously given on anything but the nursing care and the patients' well being. Working people could also pay a 'penny in the pound' of their wages into a fund, which went towards their hospital treatment if they needed it. The nurses had to ask the new admissions to the hospital if they were members of this scheme and if they were then the hospital could call on the funds available from the scheme.

The Finals, when they came around in June 1931 for me, were a longer, more advanced version of the Prelims eighteen months before. The two written papers were each one and a half hours long and theory examinations and the practical test were longer and more difficult. The time seemed to fly by for me while I was actually taking my exams, but once I had left the practical room at the end of all the many questions and tests the hours of the days until I would learn my results seemed to pass as slowly as could be. All the other nurses who were waiting for their results were in the same situation. Although we had plenty of work to do on the wards we were left on tenterhooks about our exams for the next six weeks.

I had been asked to work as a staff nurse before my Finals, which was a very great compliment to my skills, but at the time I was concerned about the strictness of the sister on the acute surgical ward, which was where I was to go if I accepted the position. My sister on the medical ward at the time I was asked about this saw how nervous it was making me and advised me just to accept the honour of being asked and worry about not being up to the job if and when it happened. "Wait," she said, "and don't cross your bridges until you come to them." I took her advice and found that the sister on the surgical ward was an excellent teacher. Her only fault, if it was one, was that she did not expect to tell a nurse twice if something needed explaining. I got on very well with her and during my wait for the Final results, she kept me too busy as staff nurse on the ward to have much time to worry.

It was traditionally a Saturday when the nurses were given their results and when the great day came, they were asked to go to matron's office one at a time. Very clean and neat, a little pale because of course there was no make-up worn at all, I stood with my hands behind my back and reported to matron. When I heard that I had passed, I was so pleased that I waited a moment, expecting matron to turn around and congratulate me on my achievement.

Matron did indeed turn around slowly in her swivel chair. She looked across her desk at me standing there before her and remarked very dryly. "Well now, Nurse Knowles, you will begin to learn!" – and I have been learning ever since.